OPTIMAL HEALTH
for a vibrant life

A 30-Day Program
to Detoxify and Replenish
Body and Mind

TIFFANY CRUIKSHANK
L.AC, MAOM, E-RYT500

I dedicate this book to my loving husband,

without his encouragement and support along the way

this book wouldn't be possible.

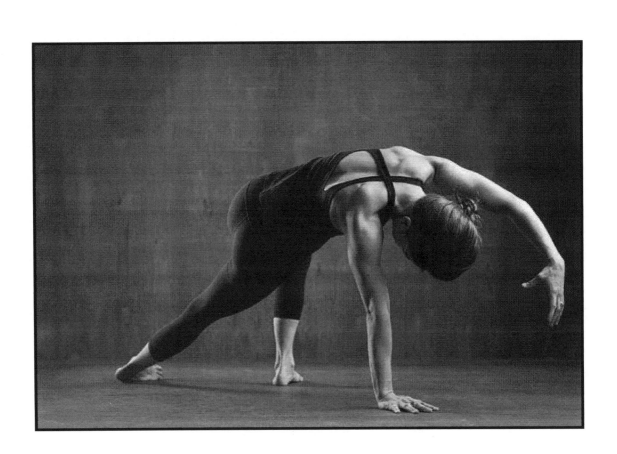

OPTIMAL HEALTH *for a vibrant life*

About Tiffany Cruikshank

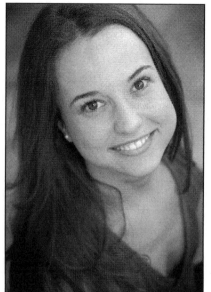

Tiffany Cruikshank has been in the holistic health field for more than 12 years, with several diplomas in nutrition and herbal medicine as well as a Masters in Acupuncture and Oriental Medicine from the Oregon College of Oriental Medicine. She is the Acupuncturist at Nike's World Headquarters in Portland, Oregon. She has founded sports medicine clinics and successfully worked with many celebrities and top athletes in New York City and Portland to refine their bodies and their health with her Optimal Health Program.

Tiffany began her studies of holistic medicine and yoga when she was just 14 years old and embarked on her first apprenticeship soon after. She has extensive training in holistic medicine, yoga, sports medicine and acupuncture orthopedics as well as contemporary medical acupuncture and biomechanics. Combining her background in yoga and holistic medicine, Tiffany created the Optimal Health Program, a system of looking at the whole body to help people achieve a personalized, vibrant state of health. Her view of health is seen through both a traditional and contemporary medical lens and her approach to medicine is both holistic and preventative. She uses a variety of methods to restore optimal health including acupuncture, hands-on manual therapy, herbs/vitamins/supplements, nutrition and yoga therapeutics.

Tiffany began teaching in 1996. She now travels internationally, leading retreats and workshops on yoga and holistic health. She combines Vinyasa yoga with a strong anatomical focus along with her background in acupuncture and holistic health to create a unique and thorough foundation for her students. Tiffany leads 200- and 500- hour Vinyasa Yoga Teacher Trainings and has also been featured in video and print ads for Nike and Lululemon Athletica.

More information can be found on her website *www.TiffanyYoga.com*.

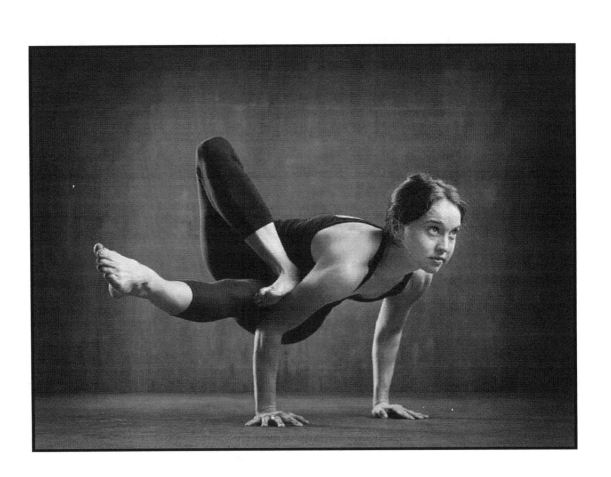

Wake Up and Live

My goal in life—and my vision for this book—is to empower my patients and yoga students to take control of their health and vitality.

In my acupuncture practice and yoga classes I often wish I had more time to teach my patients and students what they need to know to fully embrace optimal health. I began my optimal health program by working one-on-one with patients to create individualized programs for them to refine their health. Then I decided to translate these individual programs into a group setting so I could bring this information to more people. The feedback from the lectures was so positive that I decided to put it all together into a book that everyone could enjoy. The Optimal Health Program is an effective plan for achieving optimal health and peak performance, whether in athletics, work or everyday life.

Over the years I've noticed that my yoga and non-yoga patients heal differently and recover from injury or illness differently, too. As a result, I feel that yoga is a vital component of the Optimal Health Program. With that said, I also firmly believe that there is not *one style* that works for everyone but that there is *a style* of yoga for everyone. If you are new to yoga, please continue to try out new classes until you find the one that feels right to you, based on how you feel during and (most of all) after class.

The style I love and teach is Vinyasa, so that's what is mostly shown in this book. I love the fluidity of the Vinyasa style as well as its creativity and combination of flexibility, strength and stability all in one. What I show here is meant to be a guide for those with a semi-regular practice who want a more regular, home practice. The yoga instruction in this book is not meant to be a substitute for classes. Nothing can replace the guidance of a teacher's eye or the support of a group setting to keep you on track. However, a home practice can help you delve a little deeper into your yoga and create consistency and regularity. At the very least make an effort to start your day with a few sun salutations (described in Week One). You'll notice a difference in how you feel during the day.

Yoga can be a great way to reduce stress, especially when used in conjunction with good breathing techniques. Yoga is therapeutic on many levels. Physically it strengthens and creates elasticity in the tissues thereby providing a good balance between strength, flexibility and stability. Internally it stimulates detoxification and metabolism. Mentally it establishes awareness and clarity as well as a calm, confident sense of self. The beauty of yoga is that it not only addresses the physical ailments, but through regular practice it addresses our mental and emotional health and our stress levels as well. Yoga helps us develop a deeper awareness of our bodies so that we know when to push a little further and when to rest. Yoga gives us the owner's manual to our bodies so that we learn how to use and move the body more efficiently.

Thanks to more research, we are finally realizing that stress is often responsible not only for the degradation of our health but also our overall well-being. I use yoga with many of my patients for this reason. I believe it not only addresses our physical ailments, but through regular practice it also works with our mental and emotional health and stress levels, broadening the gap between action and reaction.

If you have any health concerns or physical limitations please contact your healthcare practitioner first. If you are new to yoga I recommend attending introductory classes or private lessons prior to starting this program. For the first sun salutation of the day, take a few extra breaths in each pose. As you warm up to it, gradually start to move with each breath. As we progress through the four weeks ahead, I will continue to add poses to your yoga practice, but feel free to stick to just the sun salutations or to add other poses as you like. This home practice is meant to be done on the days when you can't make it to a full yoga class. However, some people discover that they like to do the sun salutations every morning to prepare for the day, whether they're going to a class later or not.

This Optimal Health Program is appropriate for anyone: those looking to optimize an already healthy body; athletes looking to enhance their performance; or for those who need a complete overhaul. The goals—and benefits—of this program are both long- and short-term. The objective is for gradual but permanent changes that can be sustained over time. Once your body is functioning optimally, it can metabolize more efficiently for your individual needs and continue to bring positive changes for years to come. My hope is that you bring your body back to its optimal health and increase the quality of your life now and in the future.

My intention as a teacher is to awaken a new perspective of the world and to remind people to wake up and live.

Namaste,
Tiffany

How to Approach this Book

Optimal Health for a Vibrant Life is a 30-day program designed to help you detoxify your body and develop sustainable habits for a healthier future. But I'm aware that not everyone will approach this program in the same way.

I recommend first reading the Introduction and Nutrition chapters and then reading the overview for each week so you have a good idea of what you'll be doing. At this point you may already have a few things in mind that you want to leave out this time around. That's fine—don't let that hold you back from starting the program. The most important thing is to be realistic in your expectations for yourself. Plan time when you can commit to following the program to the best of your ability. If you are very busy all the time or travel a lot, don't wait for the "perfect time" as it may never happen. Just look for the best opening in your schedule in the next couple weeks.

Once you decide on a start date, write it into your calendar and make a note a few days prior so can start to prepare mentally. I want to make it clear that this program can be as easy or difficult as you want to make it. Sometimes even the simplest things can make a huge difference, but above all be honest with yourself in your needs and expectations.

I recommend buying a journal to take notes in along the way on your progress and what works for your body. You can fill out some of the questionnaires and set your goals for the week in your journal to better reuse this book in the future. You may also want to take a picture of yourself and log it in your journal so you can use it as a starting point to track your journey. It's very useful to refer to it 6-12 months later.

Each week there's an overview of the week ahead—diet, yoga, exercise, shopping and so on—that will outline everything you will do for every day of that week. Each day has a specific focus as well. If you need to cut back because you're running low on time, do so with the daily tasks first. Keep your eye on the weekly objectives.

At the beginning of each week write down your goals, making them as specific as possible. For example, you might write one of the following: "I will eliminate alcohol this week except for one glass of wine on Saturday; I will limit dairy to one serving of plain sugar-free yogurt per day this week; I will cut my caffeine intake in half every other day this week;

I will cut out refined sugar and substitute honey but continue my caffeine intake at half what I normally drink this week; or I will cut out all caffeine, alcohol, dairy, wheat and sugar for the entire 30 days."

Don't be overwhelmed by the amount of information in this book and don't feel like you have to do everything. The great thing about the depth of knowledge in this book is that you can come back to it over and over and get more out of it each time.

Yours in good health,

Tiffany

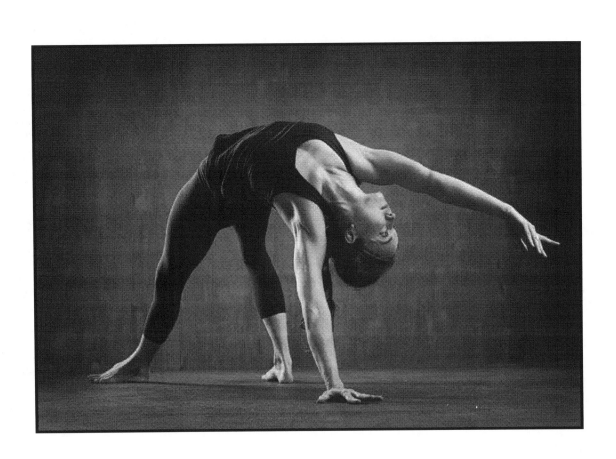

Introduction

Cleansing the mind of negative thought patterns
is essential to the detoxification process.

— page 12

What is Detoxification?

Ridding the body of toxins through a detoxification plan is an essential tool in natural medicine because of its relative simplicity, low cost and effective therapeutic results. Detoxification can be as simple or complex as needed and the effects are often immediately noticeable.

The body continuously detoxifies itself naturally, but when this mechanism is overloaded, the process becomes less efficient and symptoms like allergies, PMS, indigestion, headaches or skin problems may occur. It's important that our bodies eliminate these toxins quickly and efficiently. That's why it's a good habit to do some type of detoxification several times a year.

The 30-day program outlined in this book provides you with the tools you need to cleanse your body and mind of harmful toxins.

Detoxifying the Body

Our bodies are exposed to both internal and external toxins. External toxins like pollution or pesticides put stress on our organs to eliminate these chemicals that, as they accumulate, can wreak havoc on the system. Internal toxins like improper digestion or imbalanced microorganisms incur toxins as metabolic by-products that can further compromise detoxification pathways—even in a healthy system. However, there are many ways to minimize and eliminate these toxins from the body.

A carefully planned detoxification program can offer:

Increased energy levels

Weight loss

Anti-aging effects

Greater motivation

Better digestion and assimilation of nutrients

Better concentration and focus

Increased productivity

Reduced allergic symptoms

Clearer skin and eyes

Decrease or eliminate headaches, migraines, joint pain, body aches, colds, allergies and autoimmune symptoms, to name a few

Detoxifying the Mind

Cleansing the mind of negative thought patterns is essential to detoxification. Becoming more conscious of those patterns will add new depth to the detoxification process. It can also uncover latent emotions that create a block to optimal health by harboring unhealthy tension in the organs. It has been shown that intense emotions cause a release of chemicals that can actually keep these emotions stored in our cells so they continue to impact our physiology, sometimes for years.

Overview of the Program

This program is carefully laid out to approach detoxification in a systematic manner over the course of 30 days. Each week we concentrate on cleansing a different organ system and each day focuses on details that specifically benefit that system.

- **Week One** focuses on cleansing the digestive system. This week, too, we begin decreasing toxic substances we ingest—caffeine, alcohol and sugar. Throughout the week we look at other small changes we can make to enhance this process.

- **Week Two** focuses on cleansing the liver, our main organ of detoxification. This week we also look at some tinctures and teas we can take and other things we can do to clean up the liver. We continue to decrease substances—wheat and dairy—that can be irritating to the system as well.

- **Week Three** focuses on detoxifying the kidneys and skin. We continue to decrease the toxic load on the body by eliminating refined sugar, bread, caffeine and alcohol. This will be the most intensive week in terms of food.

- **Week Four** focuses on nourishing the body and strengthening the adrenal and immune systems. Now that we have thoroughly cleansed the body, we seek to strengthen its resilience against toxins. This week is about moderation. We develop a plan to limit—but not completely eliminate—the foods we purged from our system in previous weeks.

The last two days of our 30-day program gives guidance on moving forward after our detoxification. We also revisit our goals and priorities and make plans for the future.

Throughout the detox program, we cover many different techniques, some of which you may not feel are necessary and are tempted to skip.

Please be honest with yourself in what your body needs. Sometimes less is more, but don't fool yourself into being lazy. It's important to individualize any program as needed. However, if you are only following part of the plan, it's best to modify it at the beginning of the week when setting your weekly goals; that way you can make sure you've followed through on them. Even if all you can manage is drinking the beverages specified in the weekly overview sections, your body will still feel quite an impact.

The best part about trying out different techniques is that as you move forward after this 30-day program, you will know the effect of each technique and understand when and how to use it. As a result, you have the tools to put together your own detox plan and personalize it to your needs.

Throughout this detoxification program, feel free to pick one day a week during which you can have some limited items in moderation. That way you don't have to be a social leper to participate in detox. But remember, even on this one day moderation is key!

Now let's look at some specific nutritional guidelines. What nourishes the body and what pollutes it? What do we really need to eat?

ॐ **Yoga Instruction**

This program is not meant to be a substitute for yoga instruction but as an adjunct for those who already have a somewhat regular yoga practice, to help establish a home practice in addition to group or private instruction. If you are new to yoga, I recommend attending introductory classes or private lessons prior to this. Please contact your healthcare practitioner before starting yoga if you have any health concerns or physical limitations.

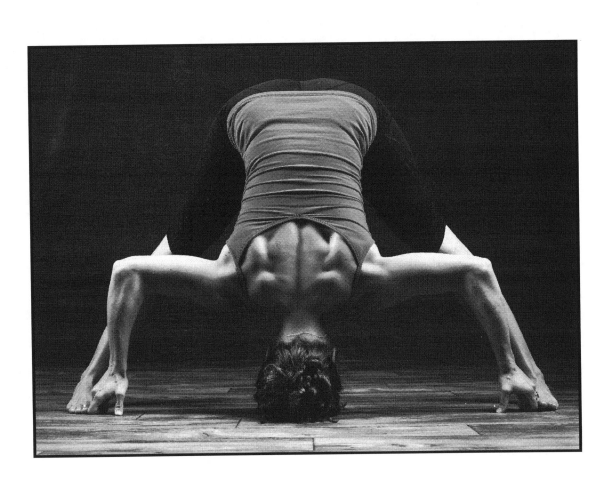

Nutrition

Your goal is not to deprive yourself or to lose weight,
but to nourish and bring your body back to optimal health
so that you can enjoy your life to its fullest.

— page 20

Nutrition: Food and Your Health

Eating a healthy diet is key to a good detoxification program. That means not only ingesting food that is good for you but also eliminating food that is bad for you. In this chapter we'll look at the building blocks of good nutrition—fats, carbohydrates and protein—as well as ways you can incorporate them into your daily diet.

General Guidelines for Good Nutrition

Because every person is so unique, I don't advocate one specific diet. Instead I advise a diet of whole foods with plenty of variety. I do highly recommend eating small meals every three to four hours to stoke the metabolic fire while not overloading the digestive system.

Usually the hardest part is making sure you get enough protein and vegetables—most prepared or prepackaged food is generally high in sugars and low in nutritional value. One trick is to cook enough food at each meal so you always have leftovers on hand to eat later or mix in with other nutritious foods.

Let's look at strategies for making each meal count.

♦ **Breakfast:** Eat breakfast with protein; cereal and muffins don't count. You must start the metabolic fire early in the day, otherwise your body starts hoarding and enters starvation mode. Breakfast supplies the nutrients for your day so choose mindfully. A smoothie is a great place to start.

♦ **Lunch:** Make a sandwich that's heavy on the insides; in other words, the inner part of the sandwich outweighs the bread part. Pile on plenty of veggies: lettuce, tomatoes, avocado, cucumber, bell peppers, sprouts, shredded carrots or beets, olives or pickles. Here's a good place to use leftover steamed veggies cooked the night before. Add some freshly cooked or leftover nitrate-free meat. Slather on a spread to add some good fats that will stabilize the blood sugar: butter, pesto, cheese, hummus or whatever spread you like to add a little flavor and moisture. Watch out for bad oils and added preservatives and sugars (read about these later in this chapter). Put it all together and slice the sandwich in half. Eat half at lunch and the other half two to four hours later. A sandwich is easy to take with you, too.

If you can't pack your lunch, order a salad with some protein in it.

In the winter I like to make a big pot of soup at the beginning of the week. Make it very simple at first and then add to it for different meals. In the spring and summer, I buy lots of fresh veggies so my fridge is like a giant salad bar.

Remember the key is to eat small portions often, using whole foods as much as possible.

♦ **Dinner:** Keep it simple. Pick some veggies and steam or stir fry them. Use coconut oil or butter when making a stir fry as these won't hydrogenate like other fats when cooking at higher temperatures. After the veggies are cooked, add a little olive oil and sea salt—unrefined sea salt should be pink or grayish in color. I like this combination with lightly cooked veggies because I can taste the subtleties of the food. You can also try lemon, honey and olive oil mixed with salt. Spices are good, too. Once you get the hang of it you can play with sauces.

Then pick a meat or meat substitute: fish, chicken, lamb, beef, tempeh or some of each. Steam, bake, barbeque or stir fry. Olive oil and sea salt are great flavorings for meat, too.

If you have time add a whole grain dish like quinoa, brown rice, millet or amaranth. Quinoa is a great whole grain with lots of protein and minerals that's quick and easy, taking only 15 minutes to cook once it boils. If you're unsure how to cook any of these grains, you can usually find instructions online. A rice cooker/steamer is very handy for cooking grains.

If you want something sweet, eat a piece of fruit an hour or two after dinner or chop up some fruit salad and mix it with unsweetened, organic yogurt. If you prefer your yogurt sweetened, use agave nectar.

Purchasing and preparing food is only part of the nutritional puzzle. Good digestion is key. Try to chew your food to a liquid form before you swallow it, which lets enzymes in your saliva predigest your food. This also stimulates the release of acid and digestive enzymes from the stomach and pancreas to aid digestion and absorption of important nutrients.

It's also a good idea not to talk too much while you are chewing your food as this interferes with optimal digestion. Limit your fluid intake with meals, too, as it dilutes gastric enzymes, making it more difficult to digest the food. A small glass of room temperature water with your meal is plenty.

Simple Rules for Optimal Nutrition

To recap, follow these general rules to make the most of your food intake:

- Eat slowly, chew your food thoroughly and enjoy the act of nourishing yourself.

- Do not eat after 8 p.m.

- Stop eating when you are 75 percent full. Give your food time to hit your stomach. If you are still hungry 30 minutes later, eat some more. Remember that you should be eating every three to four hours.

- If you find yourself craving carbohydrates and sugar, have a snack with mostly protein or fat, then wait 30 minutes. Protein and fat are more satisfying than carbs and sugar, and they are usually what your body is really craving. Fats trigger the satiety response, making you feel fuller.

- Throw away your scale. Measure your success by how you feel.

- Don't count calories. Go by how clean and nourishing your food is. Eat what you like, but use moderation and variety. Most of all get creative!

- Do not eat standing up or watching television. Sit, enjoy, relax and chew! When you do, your digestive enzymes increase naturally (by the way, thinking about food causes you to salivate and release enzymes in your stomach as well). Eating slower also helps you realize when you're full.

- Start your new food routine with a friend, roommate or family member. Encourage and check in each other.

- Learn to say "no thanks" instead of "I'm on a diet" (besides, this isn't a diet anyway).

- Make your health a priority, even with friends and family. You can't be of any use to anyone if you're not in good health. After all, you only get one body.

- Set and stick to your priorities.

How to Fuel Your Yoga Practice

Yoga plays an important role in detoxification. It cleanses impurities and restores balance to both body and mind. In this 30-day program, you'll be practicing yoga daily, so it's vital that you supply your body with proper nutrients before and after yoga.

♪ Tip: Acid/Alkaline

We are all born with a very high alkaline blood pH of 7.4; as we age this pH level gets more acidic. An acidic environment weakens the body's immune system and is believed to speed up the aging process. When blood pH becomes too acidic, hemoglobin in the blood deteriorates and the red blood cells cannot carry adequate oxygen to the tissues.

In general most grains, dairy products, meats, seeds, legumes and nuts tend to be acidic. Most fruits and vegetables tend to be alkaline. Cooked foods tend to be more alkaline than raw foods. Food's acid- or alkaline-forming tendency in the body has nothing to do with the actual pH of the food itself. For example, lemons are very acidic; however the end products they produce after digestion and assimilation are very alkaline, so lemons are alkaline-forming in the body. Likewise, meat will test alkaline before digestion but it leaves very acidic residue in the body. Soda—diet or regular—is extremely acidic with a pH of 2.5!

Before Yoga

When you do yoga first thing in the morning, practice on an empty stomach. Or you can take liquid nutrients such as a high-quality greens powder, a protein powder drink or something small/light without too much fat/protein to slow digestion. I like to have a greens powder drink before an early morning practice and a protein smoothie after. If the class is later in the morning, I drink a smoothie before yoga.

When doing yoga later in the day, eat full meals two to four hours before your practice—the time varies from person to person, based on speed of digestion and the percent of fat/protein/fiber in the food—so that your practice does not interfere with the digestive process. Have a small snack with a little protein, such as a piece of fruit and a small handful of nuts, 30 to 60 minutes before yoga to give you a steady source of fuel.

After Yoga

Replace electrolytes and water within 30 minutes after your practice. You may want to add some glutamine to help repair and rebuild muscles.

Within an hour after yoga, have a good source of protein along with vegetables to replace vital minerals, rebuild muscle and stoke the metabolic fire.

If your practice lasts for two hours or more, I recommend putting some high-quality electrolytes in your water bottle. Make sure your electrolyte replacement has plenty of calcium, magnesium and potassium as well as some sodium and a little bit of natural sugar. If you sweat a lot during yoga, make sure you get plenty of these minerals after practice. I like the Electrolyte/Energy Formula powder by Pure Encapsulations; the ingredients are high quality with a great ratio of important electrolytes for use during exercise.

Now let's look at the key nutritional building blocks: fats, carbohydrates and proteins.

Fats

Fats and cholesterol are important components of life. Fats are responsible for many vital functions in the body. They are especially important for creating hormones, such as: sex hormones (estrogen and testosterone); adrenal hormones (cortisol that regulates metabolism); and steroid hormones and prostaglandins.

Fats also create energy stores. They insulate and protect the body. They are also important components of cell membranes and provide a concentrated source of energy in the diet.

Here's a breakdown of how fats affect the body:

- **Brain:** Fats compose 60 percent of the brain and are essential to brain function, including learning abilities, memory retention and moods.

- **Heart:** 60 percent of our heart's energy comes from burning fats. Specific fats are also used to help keep the heart beating in a regular rhythm.

- **Nerves:** Fats compose the myelin sheath that insulates and protects the nerves, isolating electrical impulses and speeding their transmission.

- **Lungs:** Lung surfactant *is a lipoprotein complex that* requires a high concentration of saturated fats and enables the lungs to expand and keeps them from collapsing.

- **Eyes:** Fats are essential to eye function and are a key component of the eye's rods and cones.

- **Digestion:** Fats in a meal slow down the digestive process so the body has more time to absorb nutrients. Fat-soluble vitamins (A, D, E and K) can only be absorbed if fat is present. Fats in a meal help provide a constant level of energy and keep the body satiated for longer periods of time.

- **Hormones:** Fats are required to make hormones and the hormone-like substances called prostaglandins that are found in every tissue, cell and organ in the body.

- **Skin and hair:** Ever hear of feeding oil to a dog to make its coat shiny? Humans get their soft skin and hair from fats, too.

The distinction between adipose tissue (fat that we see in the mirror) and fatty acids (fats that we consume as a vital component of life) is important. To understand the purpose of fats and their value, we must see them as more than just a curse to the waistline.

Types of Fat

There are three main types of fat:

1. Saturated fat is found in animal fat, butter, coconut oil, palm kernel oil and palm oil.

2. Monounsaturated fat is found in avocado oil, canola oil, olive oil and peanut oil as well as almonds, pecans and macadamia nuts.

3. Polyunsaturated fat is found in fish oil, flaxseed oil, safflower oil, sesame oil, soybean oil, sunflower oil, walnut oil, corn and cottonseed oil.

Saturated Fat

Saturated fats form essential parts of all body tissues. As a result they have many beneficial effects:

• Saturated fatty acids are a major part—at least 50 percent—of the phospholipid component of cell membranes that gives our cells necessary stiffness and integrity.

• They play a vital role in the health of our bones. For calcium to be effectively incorporated into the skeletal structure, at least 50 percent of dietary fats consumed should be saturated.

• They result in lower Lp(a), a substance in the blood that indicates proneness to heart disease.

• They are useful in actually lowering cholesterol levels.

• Saturated fats protect the liver from alcohol and other toxins, such as Tylenol.

• They enhance the immune system.

• They are necessary for the proper utilization of essential fatty acids. Elongated omega-3 fatty acids are better retained in the tissues when the diet is rich in saturated fats.

• Saturated 18-carbon stearic acid and 16-carbon palmitic acid— found in saturated fats—are the preferred foods for the heart, which is why the fat around the heart muscle is highly saturated. The heart draws on this reserve of fat in times of stress.

• Short- and medium-chain saturated fatty acids have important antimicrobial properties. They protect us against harmful microorganisms in the digestive tract.

• They contain useful antiviral agents (caprylic acid).

• They are effective as anticaries, antiplaque and antifungal agents (lauric acid).

Coconut Oil

One of the most beneficial saturated fats you can consume is coconut oil.

Recent studies have shown that the fatty acids in coconut oil perform a number of essential tasks in the body.

A medium chain saturated fat, coconut oil is high in lauric acid, which is antiviral and antifungal, and caprylic acid, which is an antibacterial. Approximately 50 percent of the fatty acids in coconut fat are lauric acid, which forms monolaurin in the body. Monolaurin is an antiviral, antibacterial and antiprotozoal used to destroy lipid-coated viruses (HIV, herpes, influenza and measles as well as pathogenic bacteria like giardia, staph and strep) by disintegrating the viral envelope, thus interfering with signal transduction viral assembly and maturation. Lauric acid in virgin coconut oil kills lipid-coated bacteria but does not appear to harm friendly intestinal bacteria. The medium chain fatty acids (MCFA) in coconut oil also have antifungal properties. Not only will they kill disease-causing bacteria and leave good bacteria alone, they will also kill candida and other fungi in the intestinal tract, further supporting a healthy intestinal environment. Coconut oil is also high in folic acid, B vitamins, calcium, magnesium and potassium, to name a few.

The MCFA's from coconut oil are easily digested and absorbed, so they are put to use nourishing the body. Unlike other fats, they place little strain on the digestive system, especially the pancreas, and provide a quick source of energy necessary to promote healing. MCFA's are broken down almost immediately by enzymes in the saliva and by gastric juices, so that pancreatic fat-digesting enzymes are not necessary. This has important implications for patients who suffer from digestive and metabolic problems.

MCFA's are also sent directly to the liver where they are immediately converted to energy rather than stored as fat. Because MCFA's are easily absorbed by the energy-producing organelles of the cells, metabolism increases and the body gets a boost of energy. This burst of energy has a stimulating effect on the entire body. The fact that the body digests MCFA's immediately to produce energy and stimulate metabolism has led athletes to use them as a means to enhance exercise performance.

Cholesterol

Cholesterol is a high-molecular-weight alcohol that is manufactured in the liver and in most human cells. Over the years, cholesterol has gained a reputation as something to be avoided, but as with saturated fats, the cholesterol we make and consume plays many vital roles.

 • Along with saturated fats, cholesterol in the cell membrane gives our cells necessary stiffness and stability. When consumed in excessive

📖 **FYI: Coconut Oil**
For more information about the benefits of coconut oil, read the essay *Coconut: In Support of Good Health in the 21st Century,* by Mary Enig, Ph.D. Enig, a professor of biochemistry at University of Maryland, is one of the top biochemists in the country and one of the main scientists in this country to bring the dangers of trans fat to the public.

🍽 **Recipes:** For more ways to cook with coconut oil, see the Recipes section.

quantities, polyunsaturated fatty acids replace saturated fatty acids in the cell membrane, so that the cell walls actually become flabby.

- When cell walls soften, cholesterol from the blood is "driven" into the tissues to give them structural integrity. This is why serum cholesterol levels may go down temporarily when we replace saturated fats with polyunsaturated oils in the diet.

- Cholesterol acts as a precursor to vital corticosteroids (hormones that help us deal with stress and protect the body against heart disease and cancer) and to the sex hormones like androgen, testosterone, estrogen and progesterone.

- Cholesterol is a precursor to vitamin D, a very important fat-soluble vitamin needed for healthy bones and nervous system, proper growth, mineral metabolism, muscle tone, insulin production, reproduction and immune system function.

- The bile salts are made from cholesterol. Bile is vital for digestion and assimilation of fats in the diet.

- Recent research shows that cholesterol acts as an antioxidant. As an antioxidant, cholesterol protects us against free radical damage that leads to heart disease and cancer. This is the likely explanation for the fact that cholesterol levels go up with age.

- Cholesterol is needed for proper function of serotonin receptors in the brain. Serotonin is the body's natural "feel good" chemical. Low cholesterol levels have been linked to aggressive and violent behavior, depression and suicidal tendencies.

- Mother's milk is especially rich in cholesterol and contains a special enzyme that helps the baby utilize this nutrient. Babies and children need cholesterol-rich foods throughout their growing years to ensure proper development of the brain and nervous system.

- Dietary cholesterol plays an important role in maintaining the health of the intestinal wall. This is why low-cholesterol vegetarian diets can lead to leaky gut syndrome and other intestinal disorders.

However, like fats, cholesterol may be damaged by exposure to heat and oxygen. Damaged or oxidized cholesterol seems to promote injury to the arterial cells as well as a pathological buildup of plaque in the arteries.

High-density lipoprotein (HDL), or "good cholesterol," is one of the five main groups of lipoproteins (chylomicrons, VLDL, IDL, LDL, HDL) that transport cholesterol and fats in the blood. It is hypothesized that

HDL can remove cholesterol from buildups within the arteries and transport it back to the liver for excretion or re-utilization. A high level of HDL seems to protect against cardiovascular diseases, and low HDL cholesterol levels increase the risk for heart disease.

Low-density lipoprotein (LDL), or "bad cholesterol," is other main type of lipoprotein that you hear about. Instead of transporting cholesterol and fats back to the liver to be processed like HDL does, LDL lipoproteins transport cholesterol and triglycerides from the liver out to the tissues. Because of this, it is believed that high levels of LDL cholesterol can signal medical problems like cardiovascular disease.

Unsaturated Fat

An unsaturated fat is a fat in which there are one or more double bonds in the fatty acid chain versus a saturated fat that is "saturated" with hydrogen atoms so that there are no double bonds. A fat molecule is monounsaturated if it contains one double bond and polyunsaturated if it contains more than one double bond. The greater the degree of unsaturation (i.e., the more double bonds it has), the more vulnerable it is to oxidization or hydrogenation. Oxidation generally occurs when foods like seeds, nuts or oils are exposed to heat, air or sunlight for extended periods, which is why it is important to store your oils in a cool place out of the sun with the lid completely closed. This is also why it is important to buy oils in dark glass so that they aren't affected by light as much when transported. Hydrogenation can happen in the processing of many packaged foods or when you heat unsaturated fats past their smoking point, thereby creating trans fats.

Monounsaturated Fat

Monounsaturated fats are fatty acids with one double bond, giving the molecule one point on its structure capable of supporting hydrogen atoms not currently part of its structure. Since it only has one double bond monounsaturated fats are more stable than the polyunsaturated fats, but less stable than saturated fats and are still vulnerable to oxidation and hydrogenation.

Polyunsaturated Fat

Polyunsaturated fats are fatty acids with more than one double bond, giving the molecule two or more points on its structure capable of supporting hydrogen atoms. The lack of the extra hydrogen atoms on the molecule's surface causes it to be more vulnerable to oxidation and lowers

Why eat eggs from grass-fed or omega-3 fed chickens? It's not just humans that can't produce essential fatty acids. Animals can't make them either. So if we are to get omega-3 from animals, then the animals must consume omega-3, too. The chickens that produce omega-3 eggs are fed a diet high in flax-seeds to increase the amount of omega-3 in the yolk.

Even fish must consume omega-3 as a part of its diet; fish get their omega-3 from algae. For vegetarians the best source is directly from algae. Or we could make sure we eat plenty of algae and fish oil, why not all of the above?

the melting point of the compound significantly. This can be observed by comparing predominately unsaturated vegetable oils, which remain liquid even at relatively low temperatures, to more saturated fats such as butter or lard which are mainly solid at room temperature. This group generally has the most health benefits but also the highest risk for oxidation or hydrogenation thereby giving it the potential to have many negative health implications if not used properly.

Two Types of Polyunsaturated Fats

Fatty acids that cannot be produced by the body and therefore must be acquired through food, are called "essential fatty acids." A category of polyunsaturated fats, essential fatty acids help regulate the metabolism. The two main types of essential fatty acids that must be consumed in food are omega-3 and omega-6.

Here's a more detailed list:

- Omega-3 is found in fish oil, flaxseed oil, flax seeds, hemp seeds, herring, mackerel, purslane, salmon, sardines, walnuts, algae (E3 Live is one of my favorites) and the egg yolk of omega-3 eggs.

- Omega-6 is found in corn oil, cottonseed oil, grapeseed oil, peanut oil, safflower oil, sesame oil, soybean oil, sunflower oil, poultry and meat.

Low levels of omega-3 result in inflammation, depression, poor memory, increased susceptibility to infection, decreased healing response, cardiovascular problems, arthritis, skin inflammation, hair loss, liver and kidney degeneration, behavioral disturbances, growth retardation, weakness, lack of coordination, impaired learning ability and eventually, death. Yes, you will eventually become sick and die without omega-3. However omega-6 is easily found in the American diet in many seeds, nuts, oils and the fat of some animals so deficiency of omega-6 is very rare. Omega-3 only occurs in a few seeds and nuts (flax, hemp, pumpkin, walnuts) and fewer oils (fish oil, walnut oil). Some wild grasses and dark leafy greens have it, too.

The ratio of omega-3 to omega-6 acids is important for the synthesis of prostaglandins. Prostaglandins from omega-6 promote cell proliferation, inflammation and blood clotting, whereas prostaglandins from omega-3 do the opposite. So, for example, we want our blood to have clotting properties but we also want it to flow freely. That's why it's crucial to have a balance of omega-3 and omega-6 that is as close to equal as possible. The problem is that getting omega-3 is much more difficult.

As this chart shows, foods high in omega-6 may be deficient in omega-3 and vice versa.

Food	Saturated Fat	Monounsatu-rated Fat	Omega-6	Omega-3
Avocado (1 cup)	6 g	25.8 g	4.43 g	.26 g
Flax seeds (2 Tbls)	.6 g	1.3 g	.84 g	3.51 g
Olive oil (1 Tbls)	2 g	10.8 g	1.12 g	.1 g
Peanut butter (2 Tbls)	3.3 g	7.8 g	4.38 g	.02 g
Almonds (2 Tbls)	.9 g	6.0 g	1.86 g	.07 g
Cheddar Cheese (2 oz.)	12 g	5.3 g	.33 g	.21 g
Salmon (chinook/ 3.5 oz.)	3.2 g	5.7 g	.33 g	1.83 g
Tuna (white/ water / canned drained /172 g)	1.4 g	1.3 g	.18 g	1.6 g

What Makes Fat Bad?

Now that we've seen the good qualities of fat, let's look at the flip side. Fats are healthy when they come from whole, natural, unprocessed foods. The problem is when fats become damaged. Fats are damaged by heat, light and oxygen. High heat and chemicals used by manufacturers to process oils are the chief sources of damaged fats. One particularly damaging process is partial hydrogenation, which gives oils longer shelf life. This process creates trans fats and other altered molecules that are harmful to the human body.

Polyunsaturated fats are the most fragile. Oils that are high in polyunsaturated fats (such as flaxseed oil) must be refrigerated and kept in a dark container. Cooking with polyunsaturated fats, as well as exposing them to heat, light or oxygen, damages the fats, depleting their nourishment and creating oxidized fats and toxins. Store these oils in a dark airtight container in the fridge, use them immediately after opening and don't keep them for long periods of time. You can usually taste when they start to change.

Mono- and polyunsaturated fats are unstable, so the cooking process can hydrogenate them, creating harmful trans fats. It's better not to cook with them at all.

Trans Fat

Trans fats have been attracting a lot of media attention, but what are they exactly?

A trans fat is an unsaturated fat molecule that has been twisted and deformed during the hydrogenation process. Trans fats created through the process of hydrogenation add hydrogen atoms to unsaturated fats, eliminating a double bond and making them more saturated. These saturated fats have a higher melting point, which makes them attractive for baking and extends shelf-life. However, the process frequently has side effects. This is why saturated fats are generally much better, when used in moderation, for cooking and processing foods. Trans fats mimic natural fats in some respects, but they are unnatural to the human body and are not essential. They increase one's risk of coronary heart disease by raising levels of "bad" LDL cholesterol and lowering levels of "good" HDL cholesterol. Health authorities worldwide recommend that consumption of trans fat be reduced to trace amounts. The primary health risk identified for trans fat consumption is an elevated risk of coronary heart disease, but it has also been linked to increased cholesterol production, degenerative diseases, inflammation, accelerated aging, Alzheimer's, cancer, diabetes, obesity, liver dysfunction and infertility.

The FDA now requires food manufacturers to list trans fats on nutrition labels. If the ingredients contain partially hydrogenated oil, then the product is suspect, even if the label says no trans fats. To bypass labeling rules, manufacturers sometimes decrease the listed serving size until the amount of trans fats shown is less than .5 grams, which regulations permit listing as "zero" trans fats. No amount of trans fat is healthy.

Therefore, avoid already hydrogenated oils such as margarine and vegetable shortening as well as all products with hydrogenated or partially hydrogenated oils in them. The same is true with nuts. Because they contain polyunsaturated fats, nuts are susceptible to oxidation; as a result, nuts should not be heated, either.

With all these pluses and minuses, it's tough to figure out which fats are best to use under which circumstances. Here are your best options:

- For adding flavor to foods or for garnish, use olive oil—extra virgin, first cold pressed, organic. Drizzle it generously on top of dishes, but do not cook with it.

- For cooking, use organic coconut oil, ghee (clarified butter) or butter.

Carbohydrates

To most of us, carbohydrates are a confusing category of food. We tend to have a love-hate relationship with them. Chemically, carbohydrates are different forms of simple sugars linked together. Foods in this category include sweets, breads and even vegetables and fruits. Not all carbohydrates are created equal, however, and the body processes different carbohydrates very differently.

Let's clear up the confusion and look at the role carbohydrates play in our detoxification program.

Carbohydrates and Insulin

We all need a certain amount of carbohydrates in our diet. The body requires a continual intake of carbohydrates to feed the brain, which uses glucose (a form of sugar) as its primary energy source. However, any glucose not immediately used by the body will be stored in the form of glycogen (a long string of glucose molecules linked together). Once the glycogen levels in both the liver and the muscles are filled, excess carbohydrates are converted into fat and stored in the adipose tissue. So even though carbohydrates themselves are fat-free, a surplus of carbohydrates ends up as excess fat.

In addition, any meal or snack high in carbohydrates generates a rapid rise in blood sugar. To adjust for this rapid rise, the pancreas secretes the hormone insulin into the bloodstream. Insulin then lowers the levels of blood glucose. The problem is that insulin is essentially a storage hormone, evolved to put aside excess carbohydrate calories in the form of fat in case of future famine. As a result, the insulin that's stimulated by excess carbohydrates aggressively promotes the accumulation of body fat. When we eat too much carbohydrate, we're essentially sending a hormonal message, via insulin, to the body to store fat. The worst part is that increased insulin also prevents the body from releasing any stored fat and drives your body to use more carbohydrate and less fat, as fuel.

High insulin levels also suppress two important hormones: glucagon and growth hormone. Glucagon promotes the burning of fat and sugar, and growth hormone is used for muscle development and building new muscle mass. Insulin also causes hunger. As blood sugar increases following a carbohydrate meal, insulin rises with the eventual result of lower blood sugar. This results in hunger, often only a couple of hours—or less—after the meal.

Cravings, usually for sweets, are frequently part of this cycle, which leads to snacking, often on more carbohydrates. Not eating can make you feel ravenous, shaky, moody and ready to crash. If the problem is chronic, you never get rid of that extra stored fat and your energy is adversely affected.

◈ **Tip: Quality vs. Quantity**
Optimal health has little to do with willpower and much more to do with information. If you change what you eat, you don't have to be overly concerned about how much you eat. Adhering to a balanced whole foods regimen, you can eat enough to feel satisfied and still wind up losing fat without obsessively counting calories or fat grams. The ratio of macronutrients, protein, carbohydrate and fat in the meals you eat is the key to permanent weight loss and optimal health.

To stop this cycle you we have to moderate the insulin response by limiting—ideally, eliminating—the intake of refined sugars and grains. Insulin responses vary greatly from person to person, but generally more refined foods evoke a stronger and/or more rapid insulin reaction. Refined carbohydrates lack the natural fiber which helps minimize the carbohydrate/insulin response. Consumption of natural fiber with carbohydrates can reduce the extreme blood sugar reactions described above. Low-fat diets cause quicker digestion and absorption of carbohydrates in the form of sugar. By adding some fats to the diet, digestion and absorption is slower and the insulin reaction is moderated.

Another problem with insulin is that over time our bodies can develop insulin resistance, often known as Metabolic Syndrome or Syndrome X. If left untreated, this syndrome can develop into Type II diabetes. Here are some of the symptoms associated with Syndrome X:

- **Fatigue.** Some people are tired just in the morning or afternoon; others are exhausted all day.

- **Brain fogginess or inability to concentrate.** This includes loss of creativity, poor memory, failing or poor grades in school and various forms of "learning disabilities."

- **Low blood sugar.** This results in feeling jittery, agitated and moody. Immediate relief is experience once food is eaten. Dizziness is also common, as is the craving for sweets, chocolate or caffeine. These bouts occur more frequently before meals or first thing in the morning.

- **Bloating.** Most intestinal gas is produced from dietary carbohydrates; insulin resistance aggravates the condition. Antacids or other remedies offering symptomatic relief are not very successful in dealing with the problem.

- **Sleepiness.** Many people get sleepy immediately after meals containing more than 20 percent or 30 percent carbohydrates. This is typically a pasta meal, or even a meat meal that includes bread or potatoes and a sweet dessert.

- **Increased fat storage and weight.** For most people, too much weight is too much fat. In males, a large abdomen is more evident; in females, the hips and butt are more prominent and are frequently accompanied by "chipmunk cheeks."

- **Increased triglycerides.** High triglycerides in the blood are often seen in overweight persons. But even those who are not too overweight may have stores of fat in their arteries as a result of insulin resistance. These triglycerides are the direct result of carbohydrates from the diet being converted by insulin.

- **Increased blood pressure.** It is well known that most people with hypertension have too much insulin, and it is often possible to show a direct relationship between the level of insulin and the level of blood pressure: as insulin levels elevate, so does blood pressure.

- **Depression.** Because carbohydrates are a natural downer that depresses the brain, some depressive symptoms are not uncommon in those who consume excess carbohydrates.

These are just a few of the effects of insulin resistance. Remember there are many hidden sources of sugar in the diet today, and with this program we are starting to become of aware of what we are conditioning our body with.

Refined Sugar

Refined sugar contains no fiber, no minerals, no proteins, no fats, no enzymes—only empty calories. What happens when you eat a refined carbohydrate like sugar? Your body must borrow vital nutrients from healthy cells to metabolize this incomplete food. Calcium, sodium, potassium and magnesium are taken from various parts of the body to make use of the sugar. Many times so much calcium is used to neutralize the effects of sugar that the bones become osteoporotic due to the withdrawn calcium.

Refining means to make "pure" by a process of extraction or separation. Sugars are refined by taking a natural food that contains a high percentage of sugar and removing all elements of that food until only the sugar remains. Sugar is commonly made from sugar cane or sugar beets. After the crystals condense, they are bleached snow-white usually by the use of pork or cattle bones. During the refining process, 64 food elements are destroyed. All the potassium, magnesium, calcium, iron, manganese, phosphate, sulfate, A, D and B, vitamins and minerals are destroyed. Studies show that "sugar" is just as habit-forming as any narcotic; and its use, misuse and abuse is one of our nation's top disasters.

Glycemic Index

As stated before, not all carbohydrate foods are created equal; in fact, they each behave quite differently in our bodies. The Glycemic Index (GI) describes this difference by ranking carbohydrates according to the effect on our blood sugar levels.

⚘ **Tip: Fruit Juice**
Fruit juice is one source of sugar we often forget about. I recommend eliminating fruit juices and sports drinks. Store-bought fruit juices are frequently contaminated with mold and contain a large amount of refined carbohydrates. Each 12-ounce glass of juice has about the same amount of sugar (8 teaspoons) as a 12-ounce glass of soda, even if no sugar is added. Avoid sports drinks, such as Gatorade, because of its high sugar content as well.

📖 **FYI: Sugar and Cocaine?**
The chemical formula for cocaine is $C17H21NO4$. Sugar's formula is $C12H22O11$. For all practical purposes, the difference between the two is that sugar is missing the "N" or nitrogen atom.

(below GI 50): all beans, cauliflower, celery, cucumber, eggplant, green beans, lettuce, yogurt unsweetened, peanuts, peppers, snow peas, zucchini, tomatoes, cherries, peas, plum, grapefruit, peach, apple, pear, whole wheat spaghetti, grapes, orange, long-grain rice, green peas.

Low Glycemic Sweeteners
Agave nectar 10-19 GI, Xylitol 7 GI, Honey 55 GI.

• Low GI Foods (GI 0-54) cause a slower rise in blood-sugar.

• Intermediate GI Foods (GI 55-69) cause a moderate rise in blood-sugar.

• High GI Foods (GI 70-100) cause a rapid rise in blood-sugar.

Choosing low GI carbs—ones that produce only small fluctuations in our blood glucose and insulin levels—is an important factor in reducing your risk of heart disease and diabetes and is key for sustainable weight loss. Switching to eating mainly low GI carbs that slowly trickle glucose into your blood stream keeps your energy levels balanced and means you will feel fuller for longer between meals.

So with all that said, what does all this come back to? Whole foods!

We still need carbohydrates, but let's not throw the baby out with the bath water! It comes back to simplicity. Whole grains, as part of a whole foods diet, provide the energy, fiber, vitamins and minerals essential to life.

Proteins

Our bodies are constantly changing, constantly being broken down and rebuilt. When ingested, proteins break down into amino acids that are used for growth and repair.

There are 20 amino acids that make up all animal protein. Ten of these are essential, meaning that our bodies cannot make them, so they must be supplied by our diet. Without these essential amino acids, malnutrition quickly results because the body cannot store amino acids like it can carbs and fats. Proteins are also responsible for creating enzymes that control biochemical reactions in the body. Proteins also create the receptors on the cells that enable the cell to communicate.

But again, we come back to balance. It may be tempting to avoid carbs in favor of a high-protein diet that outlaws even veggies. Such an imbalanced diet can have serious side effects. First, proteins in extreme quantities leave a residue of ammonia that is extremely toxic, especially to the brain. Second, if we don't get any carbs, the body starts to break down muscle tissue to convert it to the glucose your body needs. We don't want to lose muscle tissue—it has a much higher metabolic need than fat. By building muscle you increase your metabolism. So to lose weight or to tone your body, you need a balance of protein in the diet.

Meat and Fish

The easiest way to make sure you get all the amino acids your body needs is to eat meat and/or fish. However, you can get them from a vegetarian diet with careful consideration to what you eat or with an amino acid supplement. But if you eat mostly whole foods, you'll get an extra dose of amino acids from the food you eat.

Although meat is not for everyone, we are lucky now to have the choice of good quality meats, thanks to the rediscovery of and reinvestment in grass-fed, free-range livestock. Up until recently, our only option was to eat meats from unsustainable farming operations. Commercially raised animals are fed estrogenic hormones to make them gain weight faster and antibiotics to increase growth rates and prevent infections due to the very close quarters in which they are confined. The residues of these drugs in our meats have a profound effect on optimal health.

Another problem with meat from grain-fed animals is that when cows eat grains their body composition changes. These changes include an alteration in the balance of fatty acids in their bodies. Grass is a cow's natural food; corn and other grains are not. Studies have shown that both the overall level of fat, as well as the level of omega-6 fatty acids, are much higher in cows and other animals whose natural diets are grass-based than those that are fed grains. Preliminary studies also show that levels of an important nutrient known as conjugated linoleic acid (CLA)—a fat that reduces the risk of cancer, obesity, diabetes and a number of immune disorders—are much higher in grass-fed animals than in their grain-fed counterparts.

Further advantages of grass-fed meat:

- Grass-fed beef is naturally leaner than grain-fed beef.

- Omega-3s in beef that comes from grass-fed cows is seven percent of its total fat content, compared to cows fed grain only.

- Grass-fed beef has the recommended ratio of omega-6 to omega-3 fats.

- Grass-fed beef is loaded with other natural minerals and vitamins.

- It's a great source of CLA that decreases the risk of many diseases.

When we switch from grain-fed to grass-fed meat, we are returning to the diet of our long-ago ancestors, the diet that is most in harmony with our physiology. Every cell and every system of our bodies will function better when we eat products from animals raised on grass.

📖 **FYI: Fish and Mercury**
The problem with fish is that over half of the U.S. electricity consumption comes from coal. As a result more than 80,000 pounds of mercury is dumped into oceans every year.

✐ **Note: Roaming Free-Range**
Farm-raised, grain-fed animals have significantly less, if any, omega fatty acids than free-range, grass-fed animals. A similar phenomenon is starting to appear in farm-raised fish.

• Whey protein shake with banana/almond butter or fruit/yogurt or banana/ fruit/egg
• Chopped fruit with yogurt (you can add whey protein)
• Boiled egg
• Apple with almond butter (you can mix in a little cinnamon and agave nectar if you have a sweet tooth)
• Salmon or buffalo jerky
• Fruit and nuts/seeds
• The other half of your lunch—save it for a snack around 3 or 4 p.m. so you don't end up eating a huge meal at dinner.

Fish and shellfish are also readily available sources of protein. Fish used to be one of the healthiest foods on the planet. However, fish is often contaminated with mercury due primarily to the burning of coal, so it is best to limit your intake somewhat. Limit your shellfish intake, too, because of the risk of viral and parasite infections. These creatures are considered scavenger animals and consume foods that may not be healthy for you.

Other Sources of Protein

Not all protein in your diet has to come from meat, of course. There are plenty of other options.

Eggs are an excellent source of protein. Organic omega-3 eggs contain a 1:1 omega-6 to -3 ratio, while commercial eggs have a 19:1 omega-6 to -3 ratio.

Soy protein comes in many forms, from unfermented raw beans to fermented tempeh cakes. In an optimal diet, fermented soy foods are preferable over unfermented products. Let's look at why this is.

Unfermented soy products are foods we've all had, most likely on a fairly regular basis. Unfermented soy foods include: fresh green soybeans, whole dry soybeans, soy nuts, soy sprouts, soy flour, soy milk and tofu. While these foods are good sources of protein, there are drawbacks to them. Unfermented soy products contain:

- Phytoestrogens (isoflavones) genistein and daidzein that mimic and sometimes block the hormone estrogen. Phytoestrogens can throw off the estrogen balance significantly and have been shown to inhibit the conversion of T4 to the active T3 thyroid hormone that can trigger hypothyroidism.

- Phytates that block the body's uptake of minerals. Phytic acid binds with certain nutrients, including iron, to inhibit their absorption.

- Enzyme inhibitors that hinder protein digestion .

- Haemagglutin that causes red blood cells to clump together and that inhibits oxygen take-up and growth.

On the other hand, fermented soy products—primarily miso and tempeh—aid in preventing and reducing a variety of diseases including certain forms of heart disease and cancers, according to many studies. Fermented soy stops the effect of phytic acid and increases the availability of isoflavones. The fermentation also creates probiotics, the "good" bacteria the body is absolutely dependent on, such as lactobacilli. Probiotics increase the quantity, availability, digestibility and assimilation of nutrients in the body (read more about probiotics in Week Three).

Peanuts and peanut butter are usually considered good sources of protein, but it's best to go easy on them. Peanuts aren't actually nuts at all, but rather legumes. Peanuts are loaded with omega-6 fats that distort the omega 3:6 ratio discussed in the fats section. They are frequently contaminated with a carcinogenic mold called aflatoxin and is also one of the most pesticide-contaminated crops.

Dairy, especially milk and yogurt, are good protein options as well. I recommend raw dairy products for the following reasons:

- Raw milk still contains all of the valuable enzymes that are destroyed during pasteurization. Without them, milk is very difficult to digest. Lactose intolerance will sometimes disappear once you start consuming raw dairy products.

- Raw milk is an outstanding source of healthy, "good" bacteria and micronutrients, including lactobacillus, acidophilus and vitamins, which are virtually eliminated by the pasteurization process of commercial milk.

- Raw milk still contains natural butterfat, which is homogenized or removed in commercial milk. Without butterfat, the body cannot absorb and utilize the vitamins and minerals in the water fraction of the milk. Butterfat is also the best source of preformed vitamin A, and it contains re-arranged acids with strong anti-carcinogenic properties.

- Raw milk does not contain synthetic vitamin D, which is known to be toxic to the liver yet is still added to most commercial milk.

- Raw milk contains healthy cholesterol.

Pasteurizing milk destroys enzymes, diminishes vitamins, denatures fragile milk proteins, destroys vitamin B12 and vitamin B6, kills beneficial bacteria and promotes pathogens. If you don't have access to raw dairy I recommend limiting or eliminating it. Instead use organic whole milk yogurt, without sugar added, in moderation.

With all of that said, it can be easy to have a negative view of food. However, it's important to remember all the positive attributes of the foods you eat as well. Use these guidelines as a base to start choosing your foods more wisely but remember how important it is to eat to nourish yourself. Remember that your food is your best medicine!

Tip: Protein Powders
Whey/Rice protein powder can help with energy and blood-sugar maintenance, especially if you're vegetarian or hypoglycemic. It can also help with cravings or detox reactions. Mix with water and drink it one to two times per day with or between meals.

I recommend a powder that's pure protein with no added ingredients or flavors; add what you like to flavor or sweeten. These are my favorite protein powders: Whey Protein by Jarrow, MediClear by Thorne, UltraClear by Metagenics. Be aware that soy protein is heavily processed and chemical-laden. Avoid it as much as possible.

Note: Many of the supplements mentioned in this book are available at www.TiffanyYoga.com.

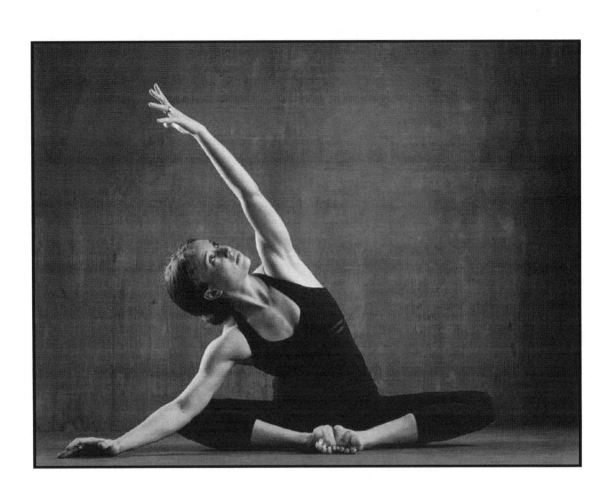

Week One

We begin to unlock an incredible potential to transform our lives
from mediocrity to greatness, where we can enjoy
and be fully present in our lives.

— *page 44*

Week One: Digest and Eliminate

This week is the beginning of our detox program and the week in which we begin to stimulate digestion and decrease the toxic load on the body. Your main objectives this week are to decrease sugar, alcohol and caffeine.

To get your detoxification underway, you'll need to do the following, every day, all week long:

1. Drink a lemon beverage in the morning.

2. Take a fish oil supplement.

3. Decrease your intake of caffeine, alcohol and sugar.

4. Start your yoga practice.

Set your goals for the week by filling out an overview chart like the one below. Make a chart like this for each and every week of your detox program. Doing this each week will help you pick and choose what you aim to accomplish that week, to individualize the program to your needs and to make those goals attainable.

Here are some examples for Week One:

Lemon drink	Daily
Sugar	Decrease refined sugar
Caffeine	Slowly transition to black and green tea
Alcohol	Only on Saturday
Yoga	Daily sun salutations, 3 yoga classes this week

Here's a blank chart to fill out for the upcoming week:

Lemon drink	
Sugar	
Caffeine	
Alcohol	
Yoga	

Let's take a closer look at each of these.

Lemon Juice Beverage. Drinking a beverage with lemon first thing in the morning—at least 30 minutes before breakfast—stimulates digestion and elimination. Follow it with a large glass of room temperature water. A quicker version is to drink lemon juice and vinegar followed by a large glass of water.

As a detoxifying agent, lemon juice can work wonders. It aids your liver in flushing out unwanted toxins, including those in the process of being absorbed into your body. It's high in vitamin C, a powerful antioxidant that boosts the immune system. Lemon juice also acts as blood purifier. When taken regularly, it serves as a tonic to the liver and prompts it to fulfill its daily digestive and cleansing functions. As a result, it helps dissolve uric acid and other poisons and also liquefies the bile. A superior alkalizer, lemon is also believed to help dissolve gallstones. Those with chronic rheumatism or gout benefit by taking lemon juice, as will those who have a tendency to bleed. Lemon is an antiseptic as well as an antiscorbutic that can prevent disease and assist in cleansing the system of impurities.

Fish Oil Supplement. During Week One you also start taking a fish oil supplement to help boost levels of omega-3 fatty acids. It's really important to purchase a good quality product that has been tested for heavy metals, such as Carlson Laboratories and Nordic Naturals. Both are reasonably priced and easy to find at whole food stores, co-ops and so on. (Vegetarians can take flax oil instead.)

Consume fish oil regularly, as it is one of the best sources of the omega-3 fatty acids that are essential to optimal health but are sorely lacking in most people's diets. Fish oil is so good for so many things, including high blood pressure, high cholesterol and dry skin. It can: lower pain and inflammation; improve memory and concentration; decrease depressive symptoms; reduce breast, colon and prostate cancer risk; and minimize ADD/ADHD symptoms, to name a few.

Decrease Sugar, Alcohol and Caffeine. Decreasing caffeine, eliminating alcohol and limiting sugar—these are very important parts of detoxification. Long term, caffeine depletes the liver, kidneys and adrenals, to name a few. Caffeine also masks our true energy levels and the ability to gauge what our body really needs. Alcohol interferes with the function of the liver, the most important organ for cleaning toxins from the body. Sugar is bad for your health in numerous ways as discussed in the Nutrition chapter.

- **Caffeine** is a powerful stimulant that, even in small doses, blocks neurotransmitters for sleep and throws off the body's natural circadian rhythm. Those who have problems sleeping should eliminate caffeine.

Furthermore, caffeine excites the adrenals that regulate stress, which are already overused and over-stimulated given our hectic lifestyles.

It's more than just its effect on the nervous system that targets caffeine for elimination from your diet. Coffee interferes with your cells' ability to use water and it quickly depletes the calcium and magnesium stores your body needs for bone health and for muscle contraction and relaxation—the contractility that releases spasms and allows muscles to stretch more like elastic and less like a wire. Coffee has been shown to raise cholesterol, impair insulin control, damage blood vessels and increase risks of heart disease, rheumatoid arthritis, stroke and miscarriage.

More than that, coffee beans are frequently grown outside of this country and are known to be high in pesticides. If you do drink coffee, drink organically grown beans to protect the health of the people working in the coffee fields and minimize their toxic exposure to the pesticides as well as your own.

If you are a regular caffeine consumer, slowly decrease your consumption. I suggest tapering your intake over the course of your first week of detox. Here's what I recommend for Week One:

Day	For those who normally consume		
Day 0	3 cups/day	2 cups/day	1 cup/day
Day 1-2	2 cups	1 cup and 1 cup tea	1 cup half caffeine
Day 3-4	1 cup and 1 cup tea	1 cup and 1 cup tea	1 cup tea
Day 5-6	1 cup half-caffeine and 1 cup tea	1 half-caffeine and 1 cup tea	1 cup white/green tea
Day 7-8	Tea only, mostly green or white tea		

This outline to decrease intake works for any substance that you consume on a regular basis and is therefore difficult to cut back. For many people the ritual of drinking coffee is the hardest part. Coffee is a drug, though, so make sure to drink plenty of water to help counteract any withdrawal reactions. Most people can avoid withdrawal side effects by following this tapering-off program; however, if you're a heavy user you may still experience some side effects—headaches being the most common—that should pass within a couple days.

• **Alcohol**—the elimination of it—is another very important part of Week One detoxification. In order to be metabolized and removed from the body, alcohol and caffeine must go through the liver. Because

✍ **Note:** For more on reasons why to avoid sugar, read "76 Ways Sugar Can Ruin Your Health," by Nancy Appleton, PhD, in the Resources section. Appleton is the author of *Lick the Sugar Habit.*

✍ **Note:** For a complete run-down about how sodas affect the body, see "Soda and Your Health" in the Resources section.

✍ **Note:** For more on the effects of sugar on your body, also refer to the Nutrition chapter.

of their priority in the liver, these products block and slow down the liver's detoxification mechanism. So it's incredibly important to eliminate alcohol during a detox.

Alcohol is also disruptive to sleep cycles, making sleep less deep and restful. It also interacts with GABA receptors and blocks the brain's oxygen sensors, complicating sleep conditions like sleep apnea. On top of that, alcohol is also a hidden source of unnecessary calories and sugars.

• **Sugar** is a substance that must be decreased, for the wellness of the immune system, digestion and cellular health and to normalize blood sugar and metabolism. This week you will to cut out refined and artificial sweeteners—white sugar, high-fructose corn syrup, aspartame and so on—as much as possible.

On average each American consumes more than 150 pounds of sugar and related sweeteners per year. It adds up quick when you consider there are 17 teaspoons of sugar in one can of cola. We often overlook many sources of sugars hidden in the foods we eat. Start checking labels so that you know exactly what you're eating. Be aware of what you're putting into your body as toxins accumulate quickly. Here are some hidden (and not-so-hidden) sources of sugar:

- Salad dressings
- Sauces (most restaurants not only use unhealthy oils and salt but usually add plenty of sugar as well)
- Condiments (ketchup, pickles, mustard, jelly, mayonnaise, tomato sauce, soup—anything canned or jarred)
- Breads and pastries
- Rice, soy and nut milks
- Juices, Gatorade, coffee drinks
- Most prepared/packaged food (snack food, frozen entrees, canned soup, packaged cereal, bread, frozen waffles, crackers)

Most of us eat large amounts of grains and sugars that generate large amounts of insulin circulating in our blood. When you stop eating these, your body takes several days to lower your insulin levels. In the meantime the high insulin levels prompt symptoms such as dizziness, confusion, headaches and generally feeling miserable. If you eat some protein and/or fiber every two hours for the first few days of your transition, you can help stabilize the blood sugar to counteract this.

As discussed in the Nutrition chapter, there are many reasons why sugar, in anything but very small quantities, is toxic to the body. Sugar over-consumption wreaks havoc with our immune and endocrine systems, leading to chronic conditions including arthritis, osteoporosis, diabetes, asthma and hypoglycemia, as well as cavities and periodontal disease.

If you drink soda, you are probably aware that each serving contains a huge amount of sugar—38-50 grams of sugar per a 12 oz. can. But sugar isn't the only problem with sodas. Phosphates leach calcium from the bones, leading to osteoporosis. Acids affect stomach juices, contributing to gastric reflux and esophageal illnesses, including cancer. Other side effects include over-stimulation and nutritional deficiencies, in addition to obesity and tooth loss.

The artificial sweeteners in diet sodas, such as Sucralose and Aspartame, carry their own risks. Studies have shown that artificial sweeteners can contribute to diabetes, Alzheimer's disease, lymphoma, birth defects and epilepsy, among others.

Now that we have an overview of what you'll be accomplishing this week, let's look at what you'll be doing each day of Week One of the Optimal Health Program.

Week One Yoga

Today you start a daily practice of sun salutations and meditation that will continue throughout the Optimal Health Program. The sun salutations are a great way to start the day; they invigorate you and prepare you for the rest of your day. After doing sun salutations regularly, you won't want to start your day without them. Sun salutations stimulate all of the internal organs and the entire musculoskeletal system as well as respiration and circulation. The meditation practice resets the nervous system so you are ready to approach your day with a calm, clear focus.

Yoga can be a great way to reduce stress, especially when used in conjunction with good breathing techniques. Yoga is therapeutic on many levels. Physically it strengthens the tissues and creates elasticity in them, providing a good balance between strength, flexibility and stability. Internally it purifies and detoxifies the organs through inversions and twisting poses. Mentally it establishes awareness and clarity as well as a calm, confident sense of self through regular practice and steady breathing. The beauty of yoga is that it not only addresses the physical ailments, but through regular practice it addresses our mental and emotional health and our stress

⚭ Tip: Artificial Sweeteners

Sucralose and aspartame can trigger or worsen:

- Diabetes
- Fibromyalgia
- Irritable Bowel Syndrome
- Chronic fatigue syndrome
- Parkinson's disease
- Alzheimer's disease
- Brain tumors
- Lymphoma
- Birth defects
- Multiple sclerosis
- Epilepsy

ॐ Yoga: Menstruation

During the menstrual cycle, women should not practice yoga for the first two days. Taking this time off is a traditional yogic practice. This is your time to rest and meditate, and to cherish your fertility! With infertility at epidemic proportions, we should celebrate this amazing power. It's a beautiful thing! Use this time to cultivate some depth to your practice outside of the asanas—for example, meditate, do pranayama, or read something inspiring.

ॐ Yoga: Nauli Technique

Nauli is another technique I like to include at the start of my practice, especially when I'm detoxifying. In this traditional practice—done on an empty stomach—the abdomen is churned left and right to stimulate the internal organs and promote detoxification and elimination.

Stand with the legs a foot apart. Bend the knees as you lean forward to rest the hands

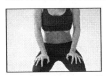

just above the knees. Place the chin on the chest then inhale deeply and exhale quickly, pressing out all the air and holding that as you draw the abdomen toward the spine. Don't mistake this for muscular engagement, like pulling in your stomach. In nuali, you soften the abdomen and then suck it back toward the spine. When you exhale completely you create a vacuum. Instead of breathing in, hold the breath and feel like you're inhaling the abdomen up into the ribs. You should be able to feel a noticeable hollow at the abdomen, no matter how big your belly is.

If you are comfortable with that, pump the belly in and out while still holding the breath exhaled. Perhaps

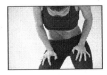

Continued on next page

levels as well. Yoga helps us develop a deeper sense of awareness of our body so that we know when to push a little harder and when to rest. Yoga gives us the owner's manual to our bodies so that we learn how to use and move the body more efficiently, without straining or hurting ourselves.

Let's get on to the poses.

1: Pranayama

We begin our practice this week with some pranayama. I like to use this breathing technique for the patience it invokes that reminds me to be present. Here's how to approach it:

♦ Start in a comfortable seated position; use a pillow or blanket to sit on as needed. We start with *Puraka Kumbhaka* in which the inhalation of the breath, its retention and exhalation will all be of equal length. Start by lengthening your inhale and exhale to a count of 6 or 8. Continue to inhale and exhale like this for several rounds. As you settle into a pace of inhale and exhale, retain the breath after the inhale. The retention of breath should be the same length as the inhale and exhale.

♦ Inhale and exhale for a count of 10 each. Repeat several times. Then inhale for a count of 10, hold the breath for a count of 10, exhale slowly for a count of 10. Repeat 3-5 times then come back to a moderately paced *ujjayi breath.*

The breath retention brings us back to the two most primitive aspects of the mind: cravings and aversions. Patanjali, who compiled what we now know as the Yoga Sutras and who is often called "the father of yoga," says every thought in its most basic form can be broken down as craving, aversion or ignorance. This breathing practice brings us back to the root of our cravings: the craving for life itself and the root of our aversions—the fear of death. As we move through this practice, we notice this craving and we soften, remembering that we're not drowning, that we're not dying but that we're examining the mind at its core and watching what happens.

The ujjayi breath calms the heart and mind and soothes the nervous system. Done gently it's beneficial for those with high blood pressure. The ujjayi pranayama technique also stimulates the Vagus nerve which kicks the nervous system into parasympathic or relaxation mode. For this reason, it's a great technique to use when you are under a lot of stress; in situations of acute stress, ujjayi pranayama stops the release of harmful stress hormones. Now we begin to unlock an incredible potential to transform our lives from mediocrity to greatness where we can enjoy and be fully present in our lives.

Optimal Health for a Vibrant Life

◆ **Ujjayi Technique.** The contraction at the back of the throat will feel similar to the sensation you get when you yawn or when you fog up a window with your mouth, except that you close your mouth and breathe through the nose. It is important to create a smooth texture to the breath to provide a soft steady base for the asanas. Relax the brain, keep the eyes soft and heavy, keep the nostrils soft and passive and keep the root of the tongue relaxed and plump. Find a brief pause at the top and bottom of the breath to instill patience in the breath and let the mind ride on the surface of the breath. Make the breath steady and even so that the inhale and exhale are the same length.

Fill the bottom of the lungs first with *Uddiyana Bandha* engaged so the abdomen stays steady but soft enough to allow the diaphragm to move. Fill the back of the body up first and then the front; make sure to breathe into the sides of the ribs as well. On the exhalation keep the spine lifting as you release the breath from the top of the lungs down.

For the full ujjayi breath count to 10 on the inhale and exhale, eventually you can add the retention. For beginners this breath will be soft and sometimes unsteady; for intermediate practitioners it is strong and steady; for advanced practitioners the breath will quiet to be lightly audible as the throat softens and maintains its steadiness.

In your practice this ujjayi breath creates a steady base to come back to. You can also use it to expand and soften into specific areas as needed. A conscious awareness will breathe life into your practice and change it from calisthenics to medicine. Eventually you will find yourself riding the breath like a surfer rides the waves, moving to the breath like a dancer moves to their music.

2: Cat/Cow (*Marjarasana*)

Cat/Cow warms up the spine by working with your breath, belly and back.

Cat/Cow (repeat 5–10 times)

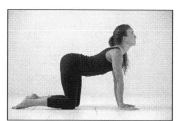 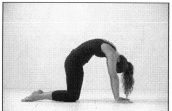 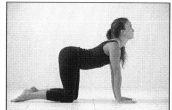

Inhale gaze up, lift chest and sit bones. Exhale round up, scoop belly, round spine and shoulders, tuck tailbone, inhale gaze up.

Continued from previous page

move the belly side to side or around in circles. Nauli tones the abdominal organs, increases the gastric fire, eliminates toxins in the digestive tract and strengthens the abdominal muscles. Nauli is best done first thing in the morning to stimulate digestion and before your yoga practice to deepen your awareness of the bandhas and the core muscles.

ॐ ***Bandha***: A breathing exercise that creates an energy lock. *Uddiyana bandha* focuses on the abdomen.

3: Sun Salutation (*Surya Namaskara*)

The Sun Salutation is an important building block in yoga as it combines a number of key asanas. For the first sun salutation of the day, take a few extra breaths in each pose. As you warm up, gradually start to move with each breath. As we progress through the weeks I will add onto this practice, but feel free to stick to just the sun salutations or even add on as you like. Home practice is meant to be done on the days when you can't make it to a full yoga class; however, some people like to do the sun salutations every morning, whether they're going to practice later or not, as a way of preparing themselves for the day.

Here are two variations on this time-honored sequence: A is the traditional sequence; B has a few more steps. Both versions include modifications with simpler poses.

Sun Salutation, Version A (repeat sequence 3-5 times)

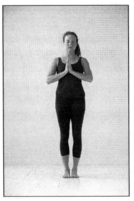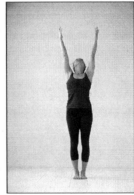

Stand in Tadasana with hands in Namaste, set your intention.
Inhale reach up, root through feet.

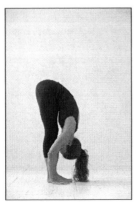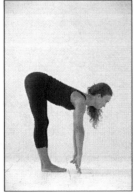

Exhale bow forward, bend knees as needed. Inhale gaze up, long spine and neck.

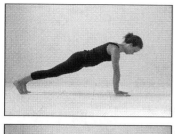 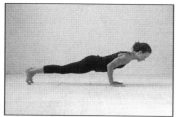

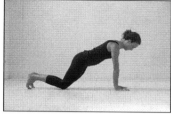 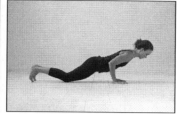

Exhale step or hop back, lift the entire front side of the body.

Exhale as you lower, elbows at 90 degrees, lift side of body.

Option: Bend knees

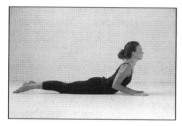 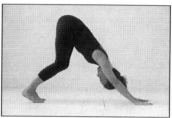

Inhale lifts the heart, shoulders roll back, thighs lift.

Exhale to Down Dog, bend knees, soften heels down, sit bones lift, shoulders away from ears, belly scoops. Take 3-5 breaths here, then inhale lift the heels and exhale, hop or walk the feet forward.

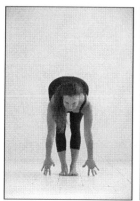 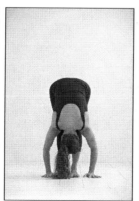 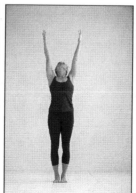 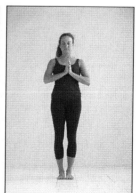

Inhale gaze up, long spine and neck. Exhale fold, bend knees as needed. Inhale lift up, root through feet to lift up. Exhale to stand. Check in.

Sun Salutation, Version B (repeat 2-5 times)

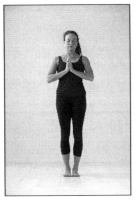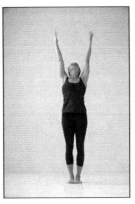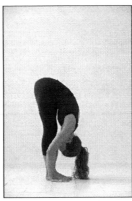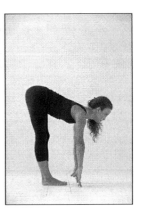

Stand in Tadasana with hands in Namaste, set your intention. Inhale reach up, root through feet. Exhale bow forward, bend knees as needed. Inhale gaze up, long spine and neck.

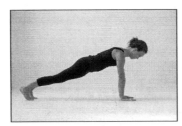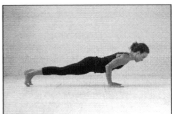

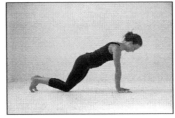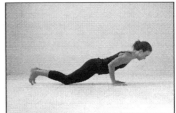

Exhale step or hop back, lift the entire front side of the body.

Exhale as you lower, elbows at 90 degrees, lift side of body.

Option: Bend knees.

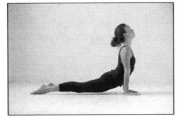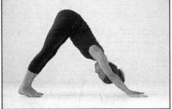

Inhale lifts the heart, shoulders back, chest lifts.

Exhale to Down Dog, soften heels down, sit bones lift, shoulders away from ears, belly scoops.

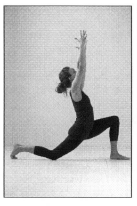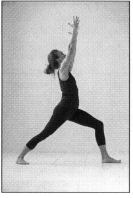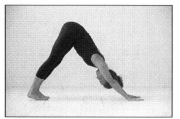

Inhale step the left foot forward, tuck tailbone, pelvis is heavy. *Option: Straight back leg.* Exhale step back to Down Dog or Optional Vinyasa.

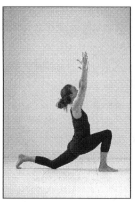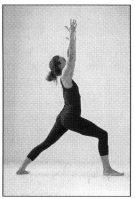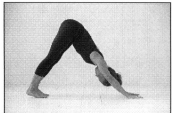

Inhale step the right foot forward, tuck tailbone, pelvis is heavy. *Option: Straight back leg.* Exhale step back to Down Dog or Optional Vinyasa. Take 3–5 breaths. Step or hop forward.

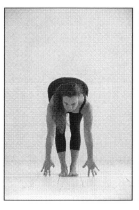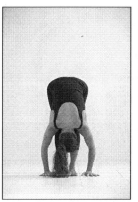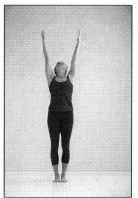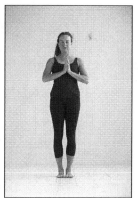

Inhale gaze up, long spine and neck. Exhale fold, bend knees as needed. Inhale lift up, root through feet to lift up. Exhale to stand. Check in.

4: Savasana

After you have completed the sun salutations, rest in Savasana—also known as corpse pose.

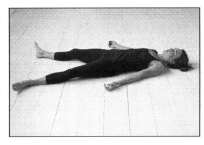

In savasana, your arms and legs are extended, with your legs spread apart a couple feet and your arms a foot or two away from the torso with palms facing the sky. After 3-5 minutes in savasana, come to a comfortable seated position on a cushion or rolled blanket. Sit and observe the natural pace of the breath.

5: Meditation (10-Count)

I often hear from people that meditation is the most life changing part of the program, mentally and physically. The meditation practices are simple techniques, but they are not easy to do or to incorporate into your life. Your mind may wander and it can be difficult to set aside the time to practice. Why set aside 5-20 minutes a day to sit and do nothing? But incorporating this or any relaxation technique into your life brings you benefits that increase over time. These include, but are not limited to, the following:

- You will lower the resting level of your sympathetic nervous system, so that the parasympathetic nervous system can conserve and restore energy.

- This in turn will regulate the heart rate and blood pressure and facilitate the digestion and absorption of nutrients.

- Your concentration will improve by strengthening the part of your mind that decides what to think about.

- You will gain increased awareness of when you are tense or relaxed, so you can calm down when you become stressed-out.

- Through this awareness, you can stop the release of harmful stress hormones that lower your metabolism, energy level, concentration and even cause premature aging.

During Week One, we start our meditation practice with a simple counting meditation. This technique is very simple and effective; however, it can be difficult to sit still at first. The trick is to keep the breath natural while you count; you'll want to control or change the breath, but instead just watch it.

Count each breath until you get to 10 and then start over again at 1. You may count to 20 or so before remembering to start over. That's OK—it's part of the process of training the mind. Just laugh and bring it back to 1. You are teaching your mind to step back and observe so you can detach from some of the constant stress and stimulus of life. Do this counting meditation for 5–20 minutes, then slowly transition into your day.

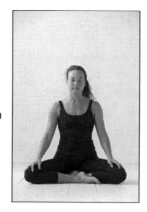

Day One

Day One establishes the foundation for the days and weeks to come. Here's the overview of what to do today:

- List your Goals and Priorities and sign the Start-up Contract: Optimal Health Program.

- Buy food and other items according to this week's dietary objectives.

- Start your daily yoga practice.

Here's the breakdown:

Contract, Goals and Priorities. Before starting any program, it's important to establish what you hope to gain and also to make a commitment to achieving those goals. Filling out the Goals and Priorities worksheets on the next pages and the Contract with yourself will help you clarify your personal intentions and motivate you to pursue them. Of course, this isn't a binding legal "contract"—no one will sue you if you don't follow through—but seeing your goals in writing may help you take responsibility for your health.

Grocery Shopping. It's always easier to stick to new dietary guidelines when you go to the grocery store with a list in hand. You'll need to purchase some items specifically for your detoxification in addition to buying fresh produce, whole grains, lean proteins and other necessities for the week ahead.

During Week One, focus on buying fresh, organic foods that contribute toward meeting the goals described above—reducing sugar, caffeine and alcohol. Because a purifying lemon drink is an essential part of Week One, be sure to add the following to your grocery list:

- 4 lemons

- Apple cider vinegar (organic, unrefined)

(Continued on page 55)

Goals and Priorities

Take a couple of minutes today to sit down and write out your goals. Then write your priorities based on your goals. Before you begin, answer the following questions. Use a separate sheet of paper so you can update your responses in the future.

1.	**What are the five things you value the most in life?**
2.	**In 30 seconds write: what are the three most important goals in your life right now?**
3.	**What would you do if you won a million dollars?**
4.	**What if you only had six months to live? What would your priorities be?**
5.	**What have you always wanted to do but been afraid to attempt?**
6.	**What gives you your greatest feeling of importance or purpose?**
7.	**What one great thing would you dare to dream if you knew you couldn't fail?**

Goals

Lifetime: When you look back from your deathbed, what will have made you the happiest?

Ten years: What do you want to accomplish in 10 years?	
One year: What do you want to accomplish this year?	
One month: What do you want to accomplish this month?	

Priorities

Fill in the chart below with your priorities, based on your goals from the previous section, then rank them in importance.

What	Very High	High	Medium
Improve my health			

Start-up Contract: Optimal Health Program

Reasons for Pursuing Optimal Health

Fill out the chart to set your intention for your health and detox program.

1.	
Why	
2.	
Why	
3.	
Why	
4.	
Why	
5.	
Why	

This contract is a commitment to myself and to my quality of my life, which means changing my life. If I am having trouble incorporating something or if doing so seems overwhelming, I will modify it in my goals for the week to make it more attainable for me or find a way to ease into the changes more slowly. I realize that at first some of these changes may seem very difficult. This is because we are creatures of habit. If I stick with making these changes, slowly over time they will become my new habits. A strong awareness of my body and mind is key to my success.

I agree to dedicate myself to incorporating these self-guided changes into my life little by little, following the outline I have been given, knowing that lasting results are in my hands. I realize that my results are dependent upon my efforts and my dedication to a long-term goal. I seek progress rather than perfection. I will review the above goals as often as needed to remind myself of my purpose. I realize that living healthy means changing my habits, lifestyle and my mind set and that it is an ongoing process rather than an endpoint.

Signature	Date
Printed Name	

(Continued from page 51)

- Honey (raw, organic)

- Cayenne power (just a little will do, 2 Tbls should be plenty)

- Fish oil or cod liver oil by Nordic Naturals or Carlson Laboratories

Familiarize yourself with your local organic markets. Usually organic produce and bulk items are cheaper and fresher at smaller stores such as food coops. Other items can be more expensive here, however.

Start refining your eye at the grocery. Shop the perimeter of the store; all the produce and fresh whole foods as well as the bulk bins tend to be found around the edges. Spend most of your time in the produce area. Buy something new and figure out how to use it.

Yoga Practice. Yoga is an important part of the Optimal Health program. On Day One begin with the sequence described under Week One overview. You'll come back to these poses again and again. You'll also learn breathing and meditation techniques that not only enhance your yoga practice but also bring a sense of calm to your day.

Day Two

Day Two is designed to help you settle into your routine as well as refine your meal choices.

- Schedule small, regular meals throughout your day.

- Continue your daily yoga practice and the weekly overview tasks.

Here's the breakdown:

Small, Regular Meals. Smaller, frequent meals or snacks with some protein and veggies throughout the day supplies a steady source of nutrition that helps stoke the metabolic fire without overloading it. When we miss meals or wait too long to eat, the body starts hoarding calories and fat, and concentration and energy suffer. As a result, we usually end up eating too much later, which strains digestion as well as the metabolism. Eat these small meals and snacks every 3-4 hours. Each of us has very different metabolic needs, some of us thrive on a higher fat and protein diet while others need more carbohydrates and still others need more of a balance. The best way to find out is to learn by listening to your body. Watch what your body tells you about the food you eat by noticing how you feel after your meal, both immediately and the next day.

Dark leafy greens (kale, chard, collards) and broccoli: high in calcium, magnesium and potassium, plus many other vitamins, minerals and antioxidants

Fruits and vegetables: bright colored fruits/veggies have more antioxidants

Whole grains (quinoa, millet, oats, amaranth, brown/basmati rice): more fiber for bowel health, as well as important vitamins and minerals that are removed in the refining process

Proteins: Fish, fermented soy (tempeh, miso), nuts, seeds, beans: walnuts and fish are high in omega-3s and are anti-inflammatory

Healthy oils: olive/pumpkin seed oil (do not cook with), coconut oil (can cook with). Coconut oil has strong antimicrobial and immune-enhancing functions. See the Nutrition chapter for more on the benefits of coconut oil.

Organic, free range, wild foods: increases the nutrient content of those foods

Natural flavors: season with olive oil/pumpkin seed oil, vinegar, citrus, herbs, touch of honey to enhance foods' natural flavors

Sea salt (unrefined): grey specks in the salt indicate minerals that benefit the body. Sea salt contains about 80 mineral elements—including trace elements—that the body needs.

This part seems easy but it takes some diligence to make sure you eat quality food. Search out whole food—preferably organic—that's easy to eat. Leftovers are very helpful here; even if there's just a little bit of food left, save it for later. Fresh fruit (whatever's in season) with some nuts or seeds or nut butter is an easy option, especially if you're on the go. The Nutrition chapter has more on this topic.

Diet Changes. Drink the lemon beverage in the morning, take fish oil supplements and decrease caffeine, sugar and alcohol.

Yoga Practice. Follow the yoga sequence described in the Week One overview.

Day Three

Day Three continues the process of settling into your routine and refining your meal choices.

- Focus on fresh, organic, whole foods.
- Continue your daily yoga practice and the weekly overview tasks.

Here's the breakdown:

Fresh, Organic, Whole Foods. Throughout Week One, you begin to refine your taste buds, which is where the lasting effects of this book will take place. We are patterned by our choices and our taste buds become accustomed to certain tastes over time. In order to have a lasting impact on your health without feeling constantly deprived, the taste buds must be fine-tuned. At first this seems difficult—because you're breaking a habit—but each week it gets easier. Diligence is key.

Eating fresh, organic, whole foods increases the nutrient content of your foods. Often our cravings for food are just cries for help from a nutrient-depleted body. Stress, caffeine, alcohol and sugar are just a few things that actually leach nutrients from the body and leave it craving sustenance.

Dietary Changes. Continue drinking lemon beverage in the morning, taking fish oil supplements and decreasing caffeine, sugar and alcohol.

Yoga Practice. Follow the yoga sequence described in the Week One overview.

Day Four

Day Four targets developing good food and emotional habits as well as continuing the work of the previous three days.

- Focus on increasing your vegetable intake.

- Generate a positive attribute.

- Continue your daily yoga practice and the weekly overview tasks.

Here's the breakdown:

Vegetables. Today, increase your daily vegetable intake by one more serving. Try adding more dark leafy greens to your diet; these are rich in vitamins and nutrients that are crucial to your health. Kale, chard and collards are good just lightly cooked in coconut oil with some sea salt. Add one more vegetable each day, every day.

Positive Attribute. Today, start paying close attention to your mental outlook. The law of the subconscious says that whatever the conscious brain dwells on, the subconscious will work to bring it to fruition. As a result, our negative self-image greatly limits our ability to change.

Take a few minutes to pinpoint one characteristic that you think would most positively affect your life. It can be optimism, confidence, clarity, efficiency, simplicity, caring, decisiveness, compassion, selflessness, etc. Then take a few minutes to sit quietly and notice, in your mind's eye, what you would look like as you go through your day with this new quality. Be as descriptive as possible. How will your interactions with the people around you change? Does your perspective of the world around you change? Do you carry yourself differently throughout your day? Notice the body language associated with the characteristic you chose. What other specifics about your day will change?

Come back to this image of yourself as often as you can throughout your day and visualize it as a characteristic that you already embody. Notice the specifics of how it changes the tasks and interactions of your day. It takes 21 days to create a new habit, so continue this exercise over the next few weeks. Keep it simple by sticking to one, clear characteristic.

Dietary Changes: Continue drinking lemon beverage in the morning, taking fish oil supplements and decreasing sugar, alcohol and caffeine.

Yoga Practice. Follow the yoga sequence described in the Week One overview.

Day Five

Keep on with your previous tasks but Day Five includes an important addition.

🍽 **Recipe: Simple Kale**

Steam or stir fry some kale. Use a little coconut oil to grease the pan if you're stir frying. Top with Lemon Ginger Dressing as described in the Recipes section.

Stress is literally just resistance to whatever the moment presents to you. Today notice what areas or moments in your day that you most resist. What would happen if you were able to let go of some of that resistance? This doesn't mean you have to stop striving for your goals, but rather that you do your best and then let go of your attachment to an outcome. Constant resistance and inner turmoil wears you down more than anything else and does nothing to help the process. What would you do with this extra energy if you were able to simply stop resisting life?

* Increase your water intake.

* Generate a positive attribute.

* Continue your daily yoga practice and the weekly overview tasks.

Here's the breakdown:

Water. Today focus on increasing your water intake. You should be consuming approximately half your body weight in ounces (for example, if you weigh 150 lb., you should drink about 75 oz. of water a day). If you sweat a lot, drink a little more than that, along with some electrolytes to replace valuable minerals lost through perspiration.

If you sweat a lot, you must replace electrolytes within 15-30 minutes after exercising—that most definitely includes yoga! When you sweat your body also releases important minerals that must be replaced. Use a low-sugar electrolyte replacement such as:

* Emergen-C powder

* Coconut water (high in electrolytes), found at most natural markets in the refrigerated or juice section, or buy a whole one in the produce section and cut it open to drink the water and eat the meat.

* Pure Encapsulations Electrolyte/Energy powder

* High-potassium foods, like avocado, cantaloupe and dark leafy greens, such as kale, chard and collards, which are high in calcium, too.

* There are many other source of electrolytes. Look for one that's not loaded with sugar and that actually has a significant amount of calcium, magnesium, potassium, etc.

Using an unrefined sea salt will help your body regulate water intake and output as well as replace valuable minerals. Make sure the sea salt you pick has pink or grey specks in it—these are the naturally occurring minerals that are taken out when it's refined (the pure white stuff). Unrefined sea salt has the same mineral profile as your blood and plenty of naturally occurring minerals to nourish your cells. So you don't need to take the same precautions you would with table salt. In fact, replacing table salt with sea salt can very easily make a huge difference in your health, especially for those with high blood pressure or fluid retention.

Positive Attribute. The law of concentration says that whatever you focus on eventually becomes your reality. Today keep your one positive attribute you defined in Day Four clearly in focus throughout your day. The power of your focus throughout this detox is as essential as your dietary changes. Don't forget to take a few minutes—maybe after your yoga practice—to visualize this positive characteristic and how it will change your day to come.

Dietary Changes. Continue drinking lemon beverage in the morning, taking fish oil supplements and decreasing caffeine, sugar and alcohol. Continue adding more vegetables to diet, too.

Yoga Practice. Follow the yoga sequence described in the Week One overview.

Day Six

On Day Six, you not only continue the work of the previous days but lay some groundwork for Week Two as well.

- Pick a tea or tincture to start taking next week.

- Generate a positive attribute.

- Continue your daily yoga practice and the weekly overview tasks.

Here's the breakdown:

Tea or Tincture. Today we will go over some choices of teas and tinctures for your liver detox next week. Whether you choose a tea or a tincture, I recommend picking 1-3 of the following herbs for your detox. To make life even simpler, you could buy a premade liver tincture that has combination of detox herbs in it. (I like Healthy Liver Tonic by Herb Pharm.)

Here are some herbs to choose from:

- **Dandelion** has many great detox functions and I highly recommend including it in your tea/tincture. If you want to keep it simple and just use one herb, dandelion is your herb: it has the widest range of uses and benefits for detox. Some of the benefits include:

  - It's a gentle diuretic.

  - It purifies the blood and liver and stimulates the manufacture of bile.

  - It decreases the amount of serum cholesterol and uric acid.

  - It maximizes the performance of the kidneys, pancreas, spleen and stomach.

Some people prefer to brew a detoxifying tea themselves while others prefer to simply buy a tincture. The benefit of tea is the process of making it and sealing your intention as you make it. Taking tea also forces you to drink some extra liquids, which also helps in the detox process.

Pick 1–3 herbs and use ½ to 1 Tbls of the dried herb (find in bulk bins at the smaller natural groceries and co-ops). Add approximately 32 oz. of filtered water, bring to a boil and simmer for 10 minutes. Then turn off the heat, cover and let sit for 10 minutes. Strain and put in a glass jar for the next day. Drink at room temperature. Sip throughout the day. Dilute with water as needed. Prepare the tea the night before the day you will take it.

✍️ **Taking Detox Tinctures**

Take 1–2 droppers of either a single herb tincture or a herb mixture three times a day, about 30 minutes before meals. If you don't like the alcohol taste, add the tincture to some warm water to burn off the alcohol. Otherwise you can just mix it with a shot of water or a small glass of water but make sure you drink a large glass of water with it.

• It has a balancing effect on the hormones.

• It's effective in treating abscesses, anemia, boils, breast tumors and liver cirrhosis.

• It may avert the development of age spots or breast cancer.

• It's of tremendous benefit to the stomach and intestines, balancing the enzymes that simultaneously benefit digestion, assimilation and elimination.

Its main actions are as a liver decongestant, liver/gall bladder stimulant, liver restorative and protective, diuretic kidney restorative and as an antilipemic, an agent in the blood that reduces high lipid levels.

• **Burdock** has the ability to flush impurities from the body with several positive consequences. It purifies the blood without side effects. The polyacetylenes in burdock inhibit the growth of bacteria and fungi, which prevents infections, especially skin infections, cystitis, colds and flu. The inulin in Burdock is a powerful immune system regulator; it is thought to attach to the surface of white blood cells and make them work better. In animal studies, inulin activated immune cells to attack cancer cells. Burdock also contains copper, iron, manganese, sulfur, biotin, zinc, iron, amino acids, mucilage and vitamins B1, B6, B12 and E.

• **Pau d'arco,** or the inner bark of the *Tabebuia avellanedae* tree, is native to Brazil, where it's traditionally used to treat a wide range of conditions including pain, arthritis, inflammation of the prostate gland (prostatitis), fever, dysentery, boils and ulcers and various cancers. In its modern use Pau d'arco is also frequently used to treat infections, including candidiasis and other yeast infections, as well as allergies, diabetes, flu, lupus, parasites and skin diseases. Preliminary laboratory research examining the properties of pau d'arco suggests that the traditional uses may have scientific merit. Such laboratory studies have shown that pau d'arco has pain killing, diuretic, anti-inflammatory, anti-infectious, anti-psoriatic and anti-cancer abilities.

• **Milk thistle** is used as a strong tonic and cleansing agent for the liver. It is so potent, in fact, that it can be used to treat liver cirrhosis, chronic hepatitis (liver inflammation) and gallbladder disorders. It's also good for:

• Lowering cholesterol levels

• Reducing insulin resistance in people with Type 2 diabetes who also have cirrhosis

- Reducing the growth of cancer cells in breast, cervical and prostate cancers

- Protecting the liver and improving its function

- **Nettles** have been used for hundreds of years to treat rheumatism, eczema, arthritis, gout and anemia. Today, many people use nettles to treat urinary problems during the early stages of an enlarged prostate (called benign prostatic hyperplasia or BPH) or for urinary tract infections, kidney stones and allergies, or in compresses or creams for treating joint pain, sprains and strains, tendonitis and insect bites. Some small but well-designed studies confirm that certain traditional uses have scientific validity, particularly in treating osteoarthritis and BPH. Surprisingly, although the nettle sting is highly irritant, once it is dried—thus neutralizing the acid—the leaves are a natural antihistamine and also have antiasthmatic properties.

- **Yellow dock** is an excellent blood cleanser and tonic. It attains its tonic properties through the astringent purification of the blood supply to the various glands and is especially useful for skin disorders, constipation and liver detox. Yellow dock also aids in the digestion of fats and oils and can facilitate weight loss due to sluggish elimination. Yellow dock is a laxative because it stimulates the flow of bile. Yellow dock root has one of the highest contents of iron in nature. This herb also balances body chemistry because of its high mineral content. It nourishes the immune system and different glands in the body. Because if its cleansing effects, it is a great endurance builder. Yellow dock is also said to tighten varicose veins as well as strengthen and tone the entire system.

- **Oregon grape root** has a distinctly bitter taste, due to the presence of alkaloids, notably berberine, which stimulates the flow of bile and therefore loosens the stools. As a result it helps prevent and relieve constipation, diverticulosis, gallbladder disease and hemorrhoids. Oregon grape also has antibiotic and anticancer properties that are receiving more and more attention by researchers and clinicians. Berberine and other alkaloids have been shown to kill a wide range of microbes and have been effective in human studies for speeding recovery from giardia, candida, viral diarrhea and cholera. It can also be used to treat inflammatory skin diseases such as eczema and psoriasis.

Positive Attribute. Continue to keep your focus on your new characteristic to make it a part of your life. Notice how you approach your day from the very moment you wake up. Your intention, whether conscious

FYI: Nettles in History

Native Americans used fresh nettle leaves to treat aches and pains. European herbalists used the leaves in a similar fashion to treat gout and arthritis. In the first century, Greek physicians Dioscorides and Galen reported the leaf of nettle had diuretic and laxative properties and was useful for asthma, pleurisy and spleen illnesses.

In Brazilian herbal medicine, the entire plant is used for excessive menstrual bleeding, diarrhea, diabetes, urinary disorders and respiratory problems including allergies. In Peru nettle is used for muscular and arthritis pain, eczema, ulcers, asthma, diabetes, intestinal inflammation, nosebleeds and rheumatism.

In Germany today stinging nettle is sold as an herbal drug for prostate diseases and as a diuretic. It is a common ingredient in other herbal drugs produced in Germany for rheumatic complaints and inflammatory conditions (especially for the lower urinary tract and prostate).

In the United States many healing properties are attributed to nettle, both the leaf and the root although for different purposes. The leaf is used as a diuretic for arthritis, prostatitis, rheumatism, rheumatoid arthritis, high blood pressure and allergic rhinitis. The root is recommended as a diuretic for relief of benign prostatic hyperplasia (BPH) and other prostate problems.

BKS Iyengar often suggests that when you find yourself trapped in negative behavior, spend more time and energy directed toward positive thoughts and behaviors. Eventually we realize that we can't beat the darkness with a baseball bat nor do we need to deny its existence. All we have to do is turn on the light. In our yoga practice we first come to know it and then we can move on, but we must focus wholeheartedly on the positive in order to bring the changes we aspire to because we will have the same degree of grace in our lives that we allow ourselves to have.

or unconscious, can make or break the rest of your day; by making it conscious you give yourself the chance to choose. Start your day today by setting your intention before you get out of bed. Notice how your day progresses as a result.

Dietary Changes: Continue drinking lemon beverage in the morning, taking fish oil supplements and decreasing sugar, alcohol and caffeine. Also, continue adding more vegetables to diet and increasing your water intake.

Yoga Practice. Follow the yoga sequence described in the Week One overview.

Day Seven

On the last day of your first week, you not only build on all that you have learned in previous days, but you also set the foundation for Week Two of the program.

• Clean your house and clean out your fridge and pantry.

• Buy supplies for next week.

• Continue your daily yoga practice and the weekly overview tasks.

Here's the breakdown:

Clean Up. Take some time today to clean your house and clean out your fridge and pantry. This is a great time to do some spring cleaning if you have the time and motivation for it. Cleaning your house and getting rid of the things you don't need can make you feel a lot lighter mentally and physically. It's difficult to have clarity when you live in a world of clutter. Our possessions can also weigh us down. Ponder what you need and get rid of what you don't. It takes time and energy just to maintain and organize all that stuff. Less is more!

Go through your fridge and pantry, carefully reading the labels, and get rid of:

• Hydrogenated oils, trans fats or cottonseed oil—any oils other than olive, pumpkin seed, sesame or coconut oil. Cottonseed oil has a high percent of saturated fats, contains natural toxins and high levels of pesticides. Organic, cold-pressed olive oil in a dark colored glass container is best and is well worth the investment. Olive oil as well as most other nut/seed oils should not be cooked with but are very beneficial when added after your food is cooked. Remember coconut oil or ghee/butter is the best for high temperature cooking.

- Any oils that are old or taste rancid. Stale oils are extremely unhealthy. When exposed to air, light and/or heat, oils oxidize. As they oxidize they become rancid, a smell detectable to the human nose. Oxidized fats can damage DNA, promote cancer, speed up aging and cause degenerative changes in tissues. Smell your oils!

- Any margarine or vegetable shortening and products made with them. Margarine has two issues: first, the process of hardening oils increases the percentage of saturated fats; second, artificially hydrogenating oil deforms the fatty acids, creating unnatural trans-fatty acids (even if the label says otherwise).

- Sugar, high-fructose corn syrup, corn syrup, any artificial sweeteners (aspartame, Splenda/sucralose, saccharin) or anything made with these

- Anything with too long of a list of ingredients or ingredients you don't know

- Anything with preservatives or artificial colors, or with MSG, BHT and BHA

- Anything that bears no resemblance to its original form

Supplies. Buy your supplies for next week, including:

- Tea or tincture of your choice (Day Six)

Optional: These items can be purchased next week, but if you want to get a jump on it, or save trips to the store, you can also get:

- Supplies for the detox lemonade (Day 10)

- Supplies for hemp/almond milk (Day 10)

- Greens (Day 11)

- Supplements (Day 13)

- Supplies for castor oil pack (Day 13)

Dietary Changes. Continue drinking lemon beverage in the morning, taking fish oil supplements and decreasing caffeine, sugar and alcohol. Also, continue adding more vegetables to diet and increasing your water intake.

Yoga Practice. Follow the yoga sequence described in the Week One overview.

Congratulations on finishing Week One! Now it's on to Week Two.

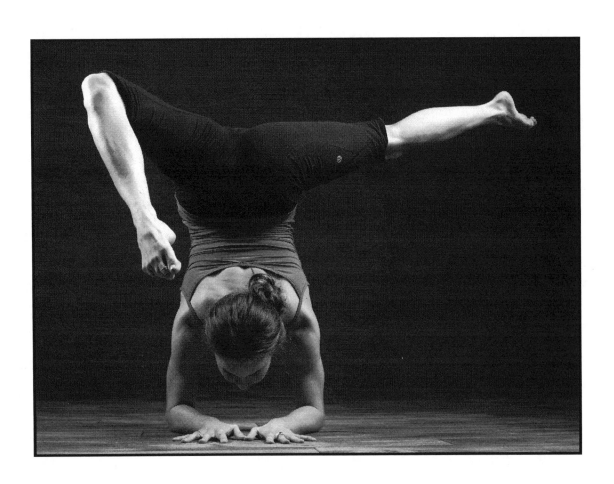

Week Two

You only get one body, one life, one chance to live

and it's difficult to enjoy your life

if you are trapped in a body

that only leaves you

sick and in pain.

— page 73

Week Two: Remove Toxins

In the second week of the detox program, we add more specific remedies to cleanse the liver. The liver is the ultimate cleanser and plays a large role in supporting the other organs. During the next seven days, you should be ingesting little or no sugar, alcohol and caffeine; you need to also decrease your consumption of wheat and dairy. Throughout this week, continue your daily yoga practice, whether at home or in a class.

You'll need to do the following, every day, all week long:

1. Drink tea or use a tincture (do this instead of the lemon drink).

2. Decrease dairy and wheat, and consume little or no sugar, alcohol and caffeine.

3. Continue taking a fish oil supplement.

4. Continue your daily yoga practice.

As with Week One, fill out an overview chart to set your goals for the week:

Tea/Tincture	
Sugar/alcohol/caffeine	
Dairy	
Wheat	
Yoga	

Let's take a closer look at each of these.

Tea and Tincture. On Day Six, you chose a tea or tincture to aid in your detox. (If you didn't do so, please choose one now.) The types of teas and tinctures and instructions for taking them are all listed in Week One, Day Six. Take your chosen tea or tonic throughout the day on an empty stomach, if possible.

Dietary Changes. In Week Two, limit dairy and wheat in your diet as well as decrease your intake of sugar, alcohol and caffeine to little or none. Here's why:

◆ **Wheat.** Most Americans consume an enormous amount of wheat on a daily basis which is why it is one of the most commonly acquired food sensitivities (along with dairy, corn and soy). Recent research has shown

📖 **FYI: Quinoa**
Quinoa originated in the Andes region of South America where it was a staple food along with potatoes and corn.

that wheat can often inhibit the normal functioning of the thyroid. Try to vary your grains by eating amaranth, quinoa, millet, oats, buckwheat or brown/basmati rice. The more you vary your food, the larger the variety of nutrients you ingest.

Quinoa is an alkaline food that is rich in amino acids and supplies a complete protein. Quinoa is especially well endowed with the amino acid lysine, which is essential for tissue growth and repair. This high-protein grain also contains many minerals and B vitamins. Those with blood sugar issues should be careful with rice as it can spike the blood sugar due to its high glycemic index. Everything in moderation.

- **Dairy.** In Chinese medicine, dairy is a mucus-forming food that, in excess, can clog your system, so consume it in moderation. This may be a hard rule to swallow, especially for women who regard dairy as their main source of the calcium that strengthens bones and thus helps with osteoporosis and other diseases. However, new research has found that high bioavailable sources of calcium come from dark green leafy vegetables (kale/chard/collard greens), nuts, seeds and whole grains.

This research has also shown that magnesium, boron, vitamin D and vitamin K are at least as important to bone health as calcium intake. These minerals not only regulate the intake of calcium into the bone, they also form the bone matrix for bone strength, improve bone mineral density and enhance calcium absorption and estrogen metabolism. The presence of magnesium in whole grains and dark leafy greens produces a balancing effect with calcium in order to regulate the contraction and relaxation of the muscles and tendons and the strength of the bones.

Yoga Practice. Continue your yoga practice as described in Week One. This week we add a couple more poses as well as new techniques for pranayama and meditation.

Week Two Yoga

This week we add some poses to stimulate and cleanse the liver and to deepen our home practice. Remember this part can be done daily or just when you can't make it to a yoga class.

1: Pranayama with Nadi Shodhanam

As in Week One, your yoga practice begins with pranayama breathing. This week we add *nadi shodhanam* in which you breathe through one nostril and then the other, alternating sides in rounds. This breathing technique helps to calm, balance and regulate both physical and subtle energies.

Nadi shodhanam pranayama offers many benefits. It helps to balance and harmonize the body and mind, thus fostering mental poise and deepening inner awareness. While practicing you are breathing deeply and consciously, which in itself warms the body, strengthens the nerves and creates stability, tranquility and clarity of mind. This practice is used to balance the two sides of the nervous system—the sympathetic that controls "fight or flight" and the parasympathetic that manages "rest and digest"—to regulate stress and relaxation. Due to the inhibiting role of stress in detoxification, this practice will assist our liver detoxification this week by calming the nervous system.

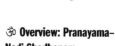

ॐ **Nadi Shodhanam**: Nerve purification accomplished through alternate nostril breathing. *Nadi* are the body's energy channels; *Shodhanam* means cleansing in Sanskrit.

ॐ **Overview: Pranayama– Nadi Shodhanam**
Inhale left, hold, exhale right, inhale right, hold, exhale left (one round). Repeat for 3-5 rounds.

To perform nadi shodhanam, cup your nose with the thumb and the last two fingers of your right hand. Place your thumb against your right nostril and your last two fingers against the left (your index and middle fingers will be folded in toward your palm). Press your thumb to close the right nostril while relaxing the fingers to leave the left nostril open. Inhale through the left nostril for a count of 5-10, hold the breath for the same count, and then press your fingers to close the left nostril and exhale on the right side for the same count.

Now do the same with the other side by keeping your fingers pressed on the left nostril, while relaxing your thumb to leave the right nostril open.
Inhale through the right nostril for a count of 5-10, hold the breath for the same count, and then press your thumb to close the right nostril and exhale on the left side for the same count. This sequence completes one round of nadi shodhanam.

2: Cat/Cow (Week One): Repeat 5-10 times

3: Tabletop with Stability work

This is a variation on tabletop with arm and leg variations to strengthen the lower back stabilizers. It is used to treat or prevent lower back pain and dysfunction and create a strong, functional core. This is great for athletes or people with desk jobs or musculoskeletal asymmetries or dysfunction.

**Tabletop Stability
(5–10 breaths each side)**

Opposite leg and arm lift, keep a long line from lifted arm fingertips through spine to lifted leg toes, belly scoops back, lifted leg inner thigh lifts to sky, long through the back of the neck

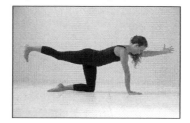

4: Sun Salutation, Version A (Week One): Repeat 3-5 times

5: Sun Salutation, Version B (Week One): Repeat 3 times

6: Triangle Pose (*Trikonasana*)

This pose is great for maintaining a healthy, supple spine while the side bending action also stimulates the liver and gall bladder, making it useful for our liver detox this week.

Triangle Pose (5–10 breaths each side)

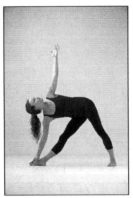 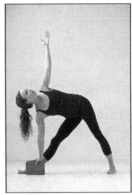 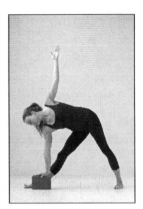

Root through feet, front ribs pull back as you lift the underside of the ribs up toward the opposite shoulder, expand through chest and arms.

Options: Use a block and/or gaze down.

7: Revolved Triangle (*Parivrtta Trikonasana*)

The benefits of revolved triangle are similar to triangle but even more potent. Though this pose may be difficult it is excellent at stimulating the liver in its cleansing and detoxification function as well as stimulating all of the internal organs and regulating the digestion.

Revolved Triangle (5–10 breaths each side)

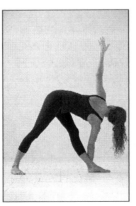 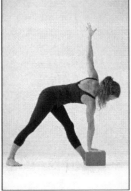

First find your foundation and square the hips to the front of your mat, then lengthen spine through the top of the head, place one hand down then rotate from the ribs, lifting the underside of the ribs up toward the opposite shoulder.

Option: Use a block and/or gaze down.

8: Boat Pose (*Navasana*)

This pose is great for strengthening the core to create a strong foundation for the lower back. It also stimulates all of the abdominal organs including the liver.

Boat Pose (hold for 5 breaths, repeat 3–5 times)

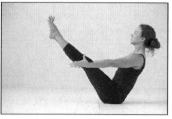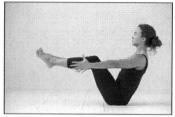

Lift the lower back off the floor, scoop the belly back toward the spine, broad chest and shoulders.

Option: Bend the knees or hold the legs with the arms.

9: Bridge Pose (*Setu Bandhasana*)

Bridge pose is a great way to learn good pelvic control and create suppleness in the spine. It is important to be mindful in this pose to maintain good biomechanics and resist the tendency to clench the glutes in toward the sacrum. Instead focus on engaging the glutes downward or think of drawing the sitting bones toward the knees while you press the feet away from the head without moving them. Remember that there is a lot of great core work just in the process of going up and down slowly so take your time. If you tend to have aches or pain in your lower back I recommend doing this pose with a block between the inner thighs to recruit the adductors to counteract the clenching of the glutes. This modification is great therapy for the low back.

Bridge Pose (stay for 1–5 minutes, repeat 1–2 times)

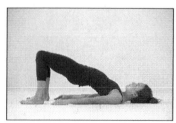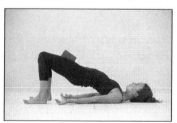

Tuck the tailbone to lift one vertebrae up at a time, feet and knees hip width apart, then come down slowly one breath at a time.

Option: Place a yoga block between your thighs.

If you are currently practicing inversions, you may add shoulder stand or headstand. Hold your inversion for 1–5 minutes, coming down as needed to child's pose.

🕉 **Yoga Index**

For a complete rundown of all poses in this program, please see the Yoga Index.

10: Twist (*Supta Matsyendrasana*)

This pose is also great for the liver as well as digestion and elimination (gas, bloating, constipation).

Twist (5–10 breaths each side)

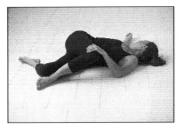 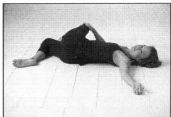

Both knees bent together or cross one leg over the other, gaze away from the knees, shoulders on the floor.

11: Savasana (Week One): 3-5 minutes

Take Savasana, then come to a comfortable seated position on a cushion or rolled blanket for meditation.

12: Meditation

Throughout Week Two, you'll practice what I call 2/1 meditation. The 2/1 meditation practice is similar to the 10-count meditation we started in Week One, but instead of counting to 10 with each inhale, with each inhale you will internally say 2 and with each exhale say 1.

I like this technique because it keeps you present without feeling like you are trying to finish something. It's easy to get caught up in the counting, like it's another thing to check off your list. While the 10-count medita-tion is a great practice to learn how to be present and notice where your mind takes you, this 2/1 practice allows you to soften a little deeper into the meditation. Starting with the 2 count on the inhale goes against the natural tendency enough to keep us present without feeling like there is an endpoint to accomplish. Continue for 5-20 minutes, take a few min-utes, then slowly transition into your day.

Day Eight

Today the emphasis is on making smarter choices about fats and looking at your exercise habits.

- Read the section on fats in the Nutrition chapter.

- Write down your exercise and yoga goals for the week, month and year.

• Continue your daily yoga practice and the weekly overview tasks.

Here's the breakdown:

Fat Education. Read the Fats section in the Nutrition chapter and start to incorporate this information into your daily eating. Update your shopping list and review the recipes at the back of this book to prepare healthier food with fats of the best quality. Eating out is another matter, as it's more difficult to closely monitor your fat intake. The trickiest part about eating out is the oil the food is cooked in. I'm not suggesting you ask the waiter what oils have been used every time you eat out; if you're eating out with friends, enjoy! But note that eating out takes its toll, even if you think you're making healthy choices.

Increase Activity. Exercise is crucial to both detoxification and optimal health; however, exercise needs vary dramatically from person to person. To find the best exercise routine for you, one that will nourish and reward you for years to come, it's essential that you listen to how your body responds after exercise, whatever type you choose. There is a deeply ingrained idea that in order to lose weight you must do cardio as much as possible, which sounds good in theory but doesn't always translate in practice. Some people need quite a bit of cardiovascular exercise while others actually do better with low-intensity activity.

What kind of exercise you need is based on how your body responds through stress hormones that alter the metabolism. I personally used to do a lot of cardio, but I didn't settle into my optimal weight and health until I switched over to yoga because of my body's tendency to release stress hormones. Granted, I do mostly Power Vinyasa yoga, which is quite active, but it also has the important stress regulation component that is key for my body.

When you are monitoring the effects of exercise on your body it is important to recognize the difference between laziness and exhaustion. When you are exhausted from working too much or exercising too much, it's best to find a mild, more nourishing form of exercise temporarily until you are able to bring your body back to health. However, if it's mostly laziness slowing you down, it's best to get yourself back into a regular routine. If it's been a while, it may be difficult to get motivated to exercise regularly. Make some goals and start small so you can progress into a sustainable routine. For many people time is the biggest issue and to that I only have one comment: you only get one body, one life, one chance to live and it's very difficult to enjoy your life if you are trapped in a body that only leaves you sick and in pain so start by creating a vibrant life right now.

Exercise can be a great stress release as long as it is something you enjoy and perceive as a release. The most important thing here is your mind set as you approach your exercise and the use of mindful breathing to reap all the stress-reducing benefits. If you are doing intense cardio it may not be possible to keep the breath deep, but try to keep a mindful observation of the breath so that even if it speeds up it stays smooth and even. Make sure that you're not tensing unnecessary body parts like the shoulders, neck, jaw or forehead. Let me reinforce this: it's not stress reduction if you are clenching, dreading it or pushing through it. Find something you can enjoy doing and be present. It may not even be the act of exercising that is enjoyable to you but more the after effects that you love. Keep that in mind so that you exercise to feed yourself rather than to beat yourself up.

Take time today to write down your specific exercise goals for this week, month and year with an honest assessment of what is realistic and what your body really needs. In yoga this is the practice of *Satya* or truthfulness and extends not only to others but also to being truthful to yourself.

Exercise and Yoga Goals for This Week		
What	How many minutes	How many times/week

Exercise and Yoga Goals for This Month:		
What	How many minutes	How many times/week

Exercise and Yoga Goals for This Year:

Dietary Changes. Continue using a tea/tincture remedy throughout the day, taking a fish oil supplement, and decreasing sugar, alcohol, caffeine, wheat and dairy.

Yoga Practice. Follow the yoga sequence described in the Week Two overview.

Day Nine

Today, notice the beauty of life around you.

- Buy some flowers for your house.
- Continue your daily yoga practice and the weekly overview tasks.

Here's the breakdown:

Flower Power. Buy some flowers for your house and place them where you'll see them often. Let the flowers be a source of inspiration to you as a reminder of all the people it takes to create something beautiful. Today as you enjoy these flowers, share your gratitude for the people around you: with someone you love, someone you don't know, someone you struggle with. Let the flowers remind you to appreciate and be grateful for everyone.

Dietary Changes. Continue using a tea/tincture remedy throughout the day, taking a fish oil supplement, and decreasing sugar, alcohol, caffeine, wheat and dairy.

Yoga Practice. Follow the yoga sequence described in the Week Two overview.

Day Ten

By now you should be feeling the effects of the dietary changes you've made. This is a good day to add some new recipes to your repertoire.

- Try some new healthy homemade recipes.
- Read about and use some of the myofascial release techniques.
- Continue your daily yoga practice and the weekly overview tasks.

Here's the breakdown:

New Recipes. Decreasing or eliminating foods doesn't mean you need to give up their flavors. For example, you can make lemonade that aids in detoxification with a sweet kick. You've already read in the Nutrition chapter—and seen in the grocery store—that options for dairy products

☯ Thought: Sweetness
As you continue to decrease your sugar intake, pause to consider why you desire this sweet flavor in your life. As in your yoga practice, seek to broaden the gap between stimulus and reaction, thereby opening a place for contemplation. Make space to choose rather than run on autopilot. Take time to breathe and delve deeply into what drives you to eat. Is it an escape? Do you eat to numb or distract yourself? Remember that to eat is to nourish your body and enjoy the act of nourishing yourself. Slow down, chew, think of all the potent nutrients you're taking in and enjoy!

FYI: Kombucha
Kombucha tea has been traced to the Chinese Tsin Dynasty in 212 B.C. In Chinese medicine it is referred to as the "Tea of Immortality" and the "Elixir of Life." Kombucha, technically a type of fungus, is popular throughout Asia as well as in Russia, Germany and Eastern Europe.

Recipe: Kombucha Tea
See the Recipes section.

are plentiful. But homemade dairy alternatives like nut milks are often simpler, more affordable and healthier than what you can buy premade. Remember to consume these alternatives wisely, however. Nut milks aren't meant to replace milk as a sipping liquid. If you're a milk drinker, fill your glass with water instead. Use nut milk to replace milk in smoothies or other recipes.

You'll find more ideas in the Recipes section in Resources.

Another addition to make to your diet, and therefore another recipe to learn, is Kombucha tea, a fermented drink that is easy to make and very nutritious. Kombucha, which is actually a type of mushroom, has a wide range of organic acids, vitamins and enzymes that give it extraordinary nutritional benefits. It contains a range of B vitamins (particularly B1, B2, B6 and B12) that provide the body with energy, help to process fats and proteins and support normal functioning of the nervous system. Vitamin C, a potent detoxifier and immune booster, is also found in Kombucha. The probiotics encourage the activity of healthy bacteria in the gut, thus restoring a healthy balance in the digestive system.

Other vital organic acids in Kombucha:

- Glucuronic acid, normally produced by a healthy liver, is a powerful detoxifier. It is readily converted into glucosamines, the foundations of our skeletal system.

- Usnic acid has selective antibiotic qualities that partly deactivates viruses.

- Oxalic acid encourages the intercellular production of energy; it's also a preservative.

- Malic acid also encourages liver detoxification.

- Gluconic acid is a sugar product that breaks down to caprylic acid to work symbiotically with butyric acid to protect cell membranes and strengthen the walls of the gut in order to combat and prevent infections and digestive issues.

Glucuronic acid, a product of the oxidation process of glucose, is one of the more significant constituents of Kombucha. It is one of the few detoxifying agents that can cope with the by-products of the petroleum industry, including plastics, herbicides, pesticides and resins. Glucuronic acid "kidnaps" the phenols in the liver so they can be easily eliminated by the kidneys. Another by-product of glucuronic acid are glucosamines, the structures associated with cartilage, collagen and the fluids which lubricate the joints.

To experience the benefits of Kombucha tea, you'll need to get a kombucha culture (as with sourdough bread, you need a fermented starter). Kombucha culture, available as a mushroom-like yeast, is fairly easy to find on the Internet. Your smaller natural groceries often carry it, too. You will need some large glass jars, sugar or honey and green or black tea.

Myofascial Release. Myofascial Release is a term broadly used to imply work on the muscles and fascia to eliminate pain and restore motion. Treatment usually uses sustained pressure into myofascial restrictions with or without movement to allow the connective tissue fibers to reorganize themselves in a more flexible, functional fashion.

Fascia is very densely woven connective tissue that covers and connects every muscle, bone, nerve, artery and vein as well as all of the internal organs. The fascial system is not just a system of separate coverings, it's actually one structure that exists from head to foot without interruption. Hence you see that each part of the body is connected to every other part by the fascia, like the yarn in a sweater. Because the fascia surrounds and attaches all theses structures, it creates a strong supportive function much like the wires of the tent that hold the tent poles—the bones—in place.

When you connect the fascia along lines of movement, our bodies are like puppets pulled back and forth by strings or lines of fascia that coordinate the muscles to work in a combined effort. Many of these lines of fascia overlap to create a multidimensional model of movement that allows us to be fully mobile. The fascia has the ability to stretch and move without restriction. However, because the muscles all go different directions they must be able to glide over and past each other. The problem occurs when the muscles and/or nerves become tethered together by bound-up fascia or scar tissue from surgery, injuries, inflammation, repetitive movements or poor posture that causes the fascia to become less pliable. It then becomes tight, restricted and a source of tension to the rest of the body. Traumas, such as a fall, whiplash, surgery, poor posture and repetitive stress injuries have cumulative effects on this fascial system. The changes these cause in the fascial system can influence the biomechanics, function and pain of the rest of the body. The fascia can exert excessive pressure, producing pain or restricting movement as well as affecting our flexibility, stability and our ability to withstand stress and strain.

Beyond that our structure can actually adapt over time to accommodate our poor movement or lack of movement patterns, so that rather than being an unchangeable bony structure we are more like a malleable piece of clay that can slowly change over time for better or for worse. This is why yoga is so crucial to optimal health, not only does it teach better posture and movement patterns, but it also teaches elasticity in the soft tissues and suppleness around the joints along with core stability and balance. When the problem is more serious, I recommend soft tissue treatments like Active Release Technique *(www.ActiveRelease.com)*, Rolfing or other deep tissue treatments that speed up soft-tissue changes. Yoga in itself will slowly retrain the soft tissue and remodel the structure of our bodies over time with mindfulness.

These myofascial release techniques are meant to help you begin to remodel your structure and to provide effects that can also supplement your physiology. For instance better posture can increase respiration and oxygen intake and therefore profusion of the tissues by this well-known therapeutic agent. Taking compression off the abdominal muscles and gently stimulating the organs can have profound effects on your ability to process and eliminate toxins. Just learning to stand upright can change your perspective enough to have a powerful effect on depression and anxiety. These and many others are reasons to be aware of the effects that your posture, exercise and mind set play in creating optimal health.

Start with the abdominal release work to stimulate the digestion, liver detoxification and elimination so crucial at this phase in the detox.

Abdominal Release

For this one you will need either a yoga block or a tightly rolled-up yoga mat or firm blanket (rolled up so that it is about 8 inches in diameter).

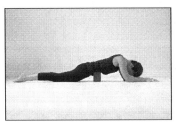 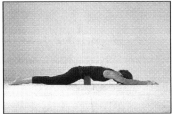

Lie on your abdomen and place the roll or block under your belly button so that it is in the soft area between the bony structure of your ribs and pelvis. With this in place come onto your forearms, take 5–10 slow deep breaths using the inhale to breathe into and expand the abdomen and the exhale to soften into the belly. Most of us store a lot of tension in our abdomen so most likely there will be some tenderness here.

If you feel comfortable here and want to proceed then you can slowly walk the hands out from underneath you to lie on your forehead. Completely relax into the belly as you continue to use the breath to guide you. This practice is inspired by Ana Forest and is a great release for the abdominal muscles and any trigger points therein as well as a stimulating pose for all of the abdominal organs assisting in digestion, elimination and detoxification.

Abdominal Release with Tennis Balls

This is a great release for tight abdominals. Even though we all love the idea of rock-hard "six-pack" abs, this area still needs to be supple as well. Trigger points in this area are often a culprit of lower back pain and can produce visceral effects on the organs as well. The tennis balls used in this technique make the pressure more specific and focused.

For this one you will need two tennis balls and a block (optional). Refer to photo for placement of tennis balls.

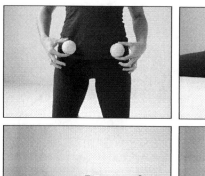
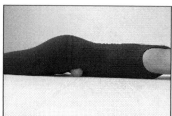
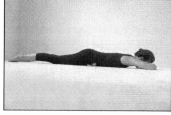
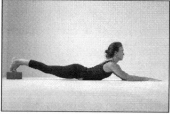

Lie on your stomach and place a tennis ball just inside of the hip bone on each side. Lay flat on the belly and relax the pelvis. If you're happy here you can lift up and rest on your forearms. For more length through the entire front line of fascia come back onto the forearms with a block behind your feet. You must pause and relax the belly completely first so that you can get into the deep abdominal muscles and hip flexors.

Then, one foot at a time or both feet together place them on the block as you reach out with the chest and maybe straighten the legs to lift the knees off the floor. Repeat with the balls next to each other just above the pubic bone then slowly make your way up the abdomen until you reach the ribs, stopping to explore tender areas along the way.

Both of the abdominal release techniques will help those with compression or tension in backbends along with the back and hip release techniques.

Dietary Changes. Continue using a tea/tincture remedy throughout the day, taking a fish oil supplement, and decreasing sugar, alcohol, caffeine, wheat and dairy.

Yoga Practice. Follow the yoga sequence described in the Week Two overview.

Day Eleven

Eliminating toxic substances encompasses more than food. Just for today eliminate television as well.

- Go on a television fast.
- Add more greens to your diet .
- Continue your daily yoga practice and the weekly overview tasks.

Here's the breakdown:

Television Fast. Don't turn on the television today. In its absence notice the space that television fills in your life and sit with the emptiness that it leaves. This is a good time to check in and see how your body is feeling. From this point forward try to minimize your television use. This is a good time to explore your purpose in life. Today start a journal entitled "My Personal Purpose in Life." Use this as a place to check in with your goals, epiphanies, struggles, realizations and your ultimate purpose for being here. Stay connected to your one positive attribute (from Day Four).

Add Greens. There are many good greens powder supplements that can help you get your daily dose of greens. I use mine as a multivitamin since the vitamins and minerals are more readily absorbed in this whole food form, but don't forget it's still important to consume vegetables as a large percent of your meals. Most greens supplements contain:

- Antioxidants to promote tissue healing/recovery
- Calcium/magnesium/potassium to regulate muscle contraction and relaxation
- Vitamins and minerals to boost energy and the immune system
- Seaweeds to help regulate the metabolism naturally
- Herbs to help with digestion and the absorption of nutrients
- E3 Live is an algae that helps to regulate metabolism, mood disorders, essential fatty acids, hair/skin health, depression, memory and aid detoxification. E3 Live comes frozen and should be defrosted each day for a 1-3 Tbls dose on empty stomach.

A green supplement can be:

- Naturally anti-inflammatory, antihistamine and an immune stimulant

- Better alternative to a multivitamin because plant-based products are more readily absorbed

- An electrolyte replacement

- A good source of natural fiber

Dietary Changes. Continue using a tea/tincture remedy throughout the day, taking a fish oil supplement, and decreasing sugar, alcohol, caffeine, wheat and dairy.

Yoga Practice. Follow the yoga sequence described in the Week Two overview.

Day Twelve

Yesterday you added greens to our diet. Today you will add more fruit, which can really help with sugar cravings in addition to being good for you! Today you will also develop a plan to establish a natural sleep cycle for your body.

- Establish a regular wake/eat/sleep schedule.

- Increase fruit intake.

- Continue your daily yoga practice and weekly overview tasks.

Here's the breakdown:

Wake/Eat/Sleep Routine. Try to wake up and go to sleep at approximately the same time every day. Eat every 3-4 hours, at approximately the same time each day (give or take an hour). Using the example below, track your hours of rise, eat and retire. Write in a specific time or hourly range at each asterisk for waking and sleeping as well as for each meal/snack.

For example:

Cycle	Wake						Sleep
Hour	6–7 a.m.	8 a.m.	10–11 a.m.	1 p.m.	4 p.m.	6–7 p.m.	10 p.m.
Food	Greens	Smoothie	Snack	Lunch	Snack	Dinner	

This pattern is really important for the body's natural rhythms, metabolism, stress, immunity, vitality and longevity. Research has shown having a regular wake/eat/sleep schedule can add years to your life.

> **Tip: Green Supplements**
> Some good green supplement options are: Earth's Promise (strawberry kiwi), PaleoGreens and PaleoReds, ProGreens, VitaMineral Greens, Ubergreens and E3 Live (blue-green algae from Oregon)

> **Tip:** Many of the supplements mentioned in this book are available at *www.TiffanyYoga.com.*

Now fill in a chart of your own:

Cycle	Wake						Sleep
Hour							
Food							

Eat More Fruit. Eat one more serving of fresh fruit a day to increase antioxidants and add fiber to your diet. Remember: moderation is key; try not to gorge on fruit, either.

Dietary Changes. Continue using a tea/tincture remedy throughout the day, taking a fish oil supplement, and decreasing sugar, alcohol, caffeine, wheat and dairy.

Yoga Practice. Follow the yoga sequence described in the Week Two overview.

Day Thirteen

While the first two steps are optional, take a moment to ponder their benefits—and then perhaps do them today!

- Consider adding new supplements.

- Apply a castor oil pack.

- Continue your daily yoga practice and the weekly overview tasks.

Here's the breakdown:

Additional Supplements. What follows are some of my favorite supplements for detox, body composition, metabolism and optimal health. Adding any of these is optional. Please consult your healthcare practitioner if you have pre-existing medical conditions or questions. I recommend adding in one or two supplements at a time so your body can better focus on their effects and then add more or switch to something different.

- **L-Glutamine** minimizes the breakdown of muscle tissue and improves protein metabolism for use after prolonged or intense exercise. Glutamine can also be taken first thing in the morning to help rebuild the lining of the digestive system. This helps maintain the gut barrier function, intestinal cell proliferation and differentiation, as well as generally reducing the symptoms of Irritable Bowel and Leaky Gut Syndrome. Glutamine also provides fuel for the immune system taken at any point in the day and can reduce healing time after surgery. Clinical trials have revealed that patients on supplementation regimes containing glutamine have improved immune and digestive function and a shorter recovery. (Take 2-4 g of Glutamine powder within 30 minutes after exercise for muscle recovery or first thing in the morning and before bed for digestion or at any time 1-2 times/day for the immune system or surgical recovery)

◆ **L-Carnitine** carries fat to cell mitochondria to be converted into usable energy, giving the metabolic engine what it needs to function properly. L-carnitine can fuel fat burning in your body, thus increasing your energy level and improving the health of your heart, your circulation and your liver. It decreases your cravings while increasing your metabolic rate. It also helps to lower cholesterol and triglyceride levels, as well as improve cardiac performance. (Take 500-1000 mg of L-Carnitine 1-3 times/day, with some food; best taken before exercise when possible.)

◆ **Alpha Lipoic Acid** (ALA) is a unique antioxidant that dissolves in both water and fat, allowing it to not only recycle vitamins C and E, but also to do the work of other antioxidants when the body is deficient in them. ALA produces Glutathione, which dissolves toxic substances in the liver. Studies also show that ALA increases Glut-4 transporters on the outside of muscle cells. This means more glucose can be shuttled into muscle cells and away from fat cells—an increase of 50-60 percent—which also makes it an excellent glucose regulator. (Take 1200-2000 mg/day of Alpha Lipoic Acid.)

◆ **L-Tyrosine** is helpful for stabilizing mood and metabolism in individuals under stress. A precursor to neurotransmitters and thyroid hormones, L-Tyrosine is an amino acid that is used by the thyroid, along with iodine, to activate the T3 and T4 hormones. Iodine (naturally derived from kelp), along with L-Tyrosine, is essential to the normal, healthy function of the thyroid gland. Supplementation of L-Tyrosine helps with stress and promotes good sleep. It also aids in the production of melanin (the pigment that gives color to hair and skin) and in the function of the adrenal, thyroid and pituitary glands. (Take 500-1500 mg/day of L-Tyrosine between meals.)

◆ **Liquid Trace Minerals** (ionic form) supply all of the important trace minerals in a highly absorbable form. You can use it like a multivitamin. (Take as directed. Sunstar Organics offers some good options.)

◆ **Vitamin D3** is essential for promoting calcium absorption in the gut and maintaining adequate serum calcium and phosphate concentrations to enable normal mineralization of bone. Vitamin D has other roles in our health, including modulation of neuromuscular and immune function and reduction of inflammation. There is so much research out there now on the importance of this vitamin, especially in the sun-restricted months of the year. Vitamin D has been found to:

- Strengthen bones
- Strengthen the immune system
- Reduce tumor growth
- Lower your risk of cancer
- Reduce your risk of multiple sclerosis
- Lower your risk of diabetes
- Decrease symptoms of Seasonal Depression

New research comes out every month about more benefits of Vitamin D3. I highly recommend this supplement. [Take 1000-5000 IU/day of natural vitamin D3 (cholecalciferol).]

- **Bladderwrack,** or kelp, is useful in the treatment of underactive thyroid glands. People who are overweight due to thyroid trouble may benefit from kelp's biologically active iodine that helps to maintain a healthy thyroid. Bladderwrack has long been used to soothe irritated and inflamed tissues in the body and can be used for constipation, diarrhea, gastritis, gastroesophageal reflux disease (GERD), heartburn, hypothyroidism, indigestion, iodine deficiency and topical wound healing. It's reputed to relieve rheumatism and rheumatoid arthritis and to exert anti-estrogenic effects in pre-menopausal women. Studies also suggest that seaweed may be an important dietary component that is responsible for the reduced risk of estrogen-related cancers observed in Japanese populations. (Take 500 mg/day of Bladderwrack, between meals.)

- **L-Theanine** helps with stress and tension (take 200 mg 3 times/day with or between meals) and aids sleep. (Take 200-400 mg 1 hour before bed.)

- **Apple cider vinegar** stimulates stomach acid and digestive enzymes. (Take 1 Tbls, 5-10 minutes before meals.)

- **E3 Live** is an algae that helps to regulate metabolism, mood disorders, essential fatty acids, hair/skin health, depression, memory and aid detoxification. (Take 1-3 Tbls/day of E3 Live on empty stomach.

- **Magnesium** helps regulate muscle contraction and relaxation for muscle cramps and spasms. It regulates blood pressure and cholesterol and strengthens the bones by improving bone mineral density. Magnesium plays an important role in carbohydrate metabolism as it influences the release and activity of cortisol and insulin, the hormone that helps control blood glucose sugar levels. It also helps support the adrenals, production of hormones, regulates nerve conduction by maintaining the myelin sheath around the nerves, activates vitamins C and E, and is used for protein synthesis. Magnesium Glycinate is the only form that won't cause diarrhea if you are sensitive to this or taking higher doses. (Take 300-600 mg/day of magnesium, with or between meals

- **Similase** and Similase BV ("BV" stands for beans and veggies) are enzymes that aid in digestion. (Take 1-2 pills, 5-10 minutess prior to meals or with meals.)

- **Vitamin B Complex** improves energy levels, nerve conduction, concentration and so much more! This is another supplement I recommend for general health since it is easily depleted with stress, caffeine and alcohol. Your supplement should have at least 100 mg or mcgs of each of the B vitamins. (Follow the dose information on the bottle, usually it's one pill, with food.)

Castor Oil Pack. While it's an optional step in this program, using a castor oil pack is a great way to deepen your detoxification. Applied as a pack placed over the abdomen, the oil of the castor bean (*Oleum ricini* or Palma Christi) is absorbed to provide a cleansing, nutritive and relaxing treatment. I highly recommend a castor oil pack when you eliminate a food or substance from your diet, especially sugar or coffee. It often eliminates the symptoms of withdrawal, such as headache and irritability. Using a castor oil pack is a powerful liver detox technique and also improves assimilation of nutrients, facilitates elimination through the digestive and urinary tract, reduces inflammation and increases circulation of blood and lymphatic fluid. Preliminary studies on castor oil packs done at the George Washington School of Medicine also indicate improved immune function.

- **Making a Castor Oil Pack.** Supplies needed:
    - Castor oil (small or medium sized bottle)
    - Plastic sheet (can use plastic wrap or trash bag)
    - 1- to 2-foot square of white cotton, flannel or wool

✒ Tip: Pregnancy Precaution
Castor oil packs should not be used while pregnant, bleeding or during menstruation.

- Heating pad or hot water bottle

- Large old towel or sheet and a rag for hands

- Old blanket

1. Prepare the surface you'll be lying on. Lay down an old blanket, covered by an old towel or sheet. On top of that put down a large sheet of plastic. These will hold in heat and prevent staining.

2. Lie on your back and carefully pour a few tablespoons of oil onto the abdomen (enough to cover it) then place the cotton or wool sheet on top and soak it as well by pouring on more oil. This oil-soaked material is the "pack."

3. Wrap yourself in the plastic piece and place a heating pad or hot water bottle on top of the plastic over your abdomen. Wrap the towel and wool blanket on top with the arms free.

4. Stay for 30-90 minutes.

5. After you've unwrapped yourself, use the rag to wipe the oil off.

6. Reuse the oil and cloth pack several times. Add more oil as needed to keep the cloth well saturated. Replace the entire pack after it begins to change color. This may occur in days, weeks or even months.

The castor oil pack will be most effective when left on for 30-90 minutes and done for 4 or 5 consecutive days per week. A castor oil treatment can be done once as a detox or more regularly for therapeutic uses.

Dietary Changes. Continue using a tea/tincture remedy throughout the day, taking a fish oil supplement, and decreasing sugar, alcohol, caffeine, wheat and dairy.

Yoga Practice. Follow the yoga sequence described in the Week Two overview.

Day Fourteen

As you end Week Two, today get a breath of fresh air to prepare for the week ahead.

- Spend some time out in nature today.

- Buy supplies for next week.

- Continue your daily yoga practice and the weekly overview tasks.

Here's the breakdown:

Mother Nature. Find time today to get out in nature, even if it's just a walk in your local park. Get out, breathe and enjoy the beauty all around you! No expectations, no destination, nothing to accomplish. Just be.

When you do your sun salutations today make them an offering, maybe even dedicate your practice to someone or something.

Go Shopping. Buy supplies for next week:

- Pure organic unsweetened cranberry juice (two 32 oz. jars—glass only)
- Lots of good whole foods without sugar, alcohol, caffeine, wheat or dairy.

Optional purchases:

- Dry skin brush and/or supplies for hydrotherapy of your choice (Day 17)
- Set up a massage or acupuncture appointment for next week (Day 19)
- Supplies for foot bath of your choice (Day 20)

Dietary Changes. Continue using a tea/tincture remedy throughout the day, taking a fish oil supplement, and decreasing sugar, alcohol, caffeine, wheat and dairy.

Yoga Practice. Follow the yoga sequence described in the Week Two overview.

You're halfway through your Optimal Health detoxification program. Let's move on to Week Three.

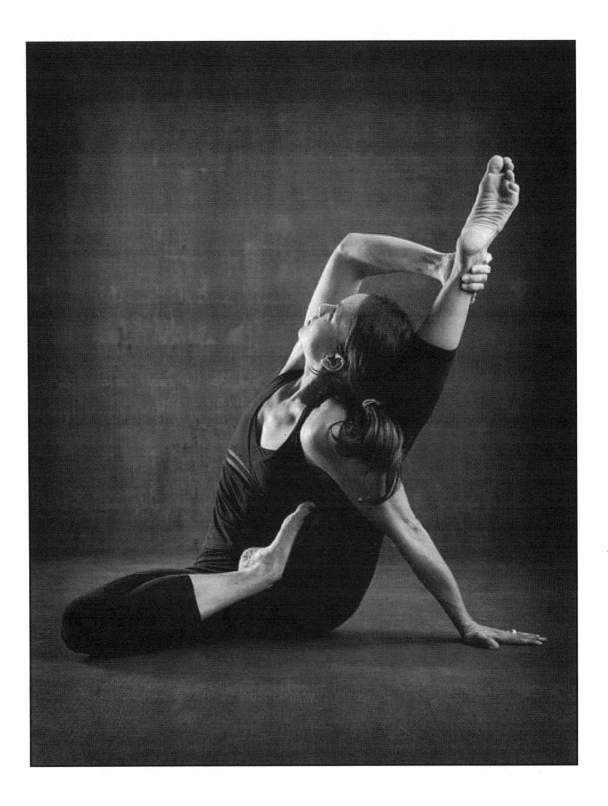

Week Three

As you approach your yoga practice,
make it an act of appreciation
for your body and health.

—*page 107*

Week Three: Clear Fluids

In this third week of our optimal health and detox program, we focus on cleansing and revitalizing the kidneys and skin. At this point, you should be consuming little or no sugar, alcohol, caffeine, wheat and dairy. Throughout this week, continue your daily yoga practice whether it's at home or in a class.

Here is what you'll be doing all week long:

1. Drink the cranberry beverage.

2. Consume little or no sugar, alcohol, caffeine, wheat and dairy.

3. Continue your daily yoga practice and meditation this week.

As with the previous weeks, fill out an overview chart to set your goals for the week:

Cranberry drink	
Sugar/caffeine/alcohol	
Dairy/wheat	
Yoga	

Let's take a closer look at each of these.

Cranberry Drink. Each day drink a mix of water and pure organic unsweetened cranberry juice. Combine 8 oz. of cranberry juice with 24 oz. of filtered water and sip it throughout the day. Drink this in addition to your normal water intake (half your body weight in ounces).

Dietary Changes. Notice your attachment to caffeine, sugar and bread this week. As you eliminate them, notice that you have a more accurate gauge of your real energy level, so that you can pace and take care of yourself accordingly, rather than waiting until you hit the end of your reserves and find yourself completely tapped out or sick and forced to listen to your body.

My beef with caffeine is that it separates me from reality, leaving me feeling like I could go forever when my body may be crying out for something else. The other issue is that even though caffeine initially suppresses the appetite, its rebound effect leaves you starving hours later when you realize you've waited too long to eat and as a result have an uncontrollable appetite. Then you gorge and feel stuffed and uncomfortable. This cycle makes it difficult to eat small meals frequently as suggested by this detox program. This week try your life without caffeine and sugar, difficult as it may be. Consider it a practice of *Satya*, or truth, which is the second *yama* in the Eight Limbs of Yoga. Use this truthfulness to see the reality of what your body is asking for and sit with that recognition to uncover your inner radiance.

Yoga Practice. Continue your yoga practice this week, adding a couple more poses and some new pranayama and meditation techniques.

Week Three Yoga

1: Viloma Pranayama

Viloma pranayama is a practice of patience and contentment, resting the nerves and calming the brain. When done lying down it is used for fatigue, weakness or strain. When seated it is said to create exhilaration, endurance and calmness.

Start with several rounds of ujjayi pranayama. Exhale completely. Inhale a third of the way and hold briefly, then inhale two thirds and hold briefly, lastly inhale completely and hold. Exhale slowly and repeat 3-5 times. Then continue ujjayi pranayama for several rounds.

2: Cat/Cow (Week One): Repeat 5-10 times

3: Tabletop Stability (Week One): Hold for 5-10 breaths each side

4: Sun Salutation, Version A (Week One): Repeat 3-5 times

5: Sun Salutation, Version B (Week One): Repeat 5 times

6: Triangle Pose (Week Two): Hold for 5-10 breaths each side

7: Revolved Triangle (Week Two): Hold for 5-10 breaths each side

8: Extended Side Angle Pose (*Utthita Parsvakonasana*)

This is another great pose to stimulate the liver and digestive organs as well as the kidneys. This pose, along with all the standing poses, is great for learning stability of body and mind.

Extended Side Angle Pose (5–10 breaths each side)

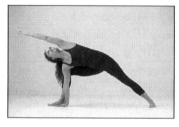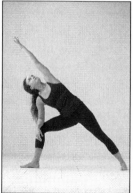

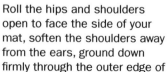

Roll the hips and shoulders open to face the side of your mat, soften the shoulders away from the ears, ground down firmly through the outer edge of the straight-leg foot to lift the inner thigh toward the bone, roll the chest open toward the sky, lift the underside of the ribs up toward the opposite shoulder.

Option: Rest your arm on your knee.

9: Locust Pose (*Salabhasana*)

This pose is great for toning the kidneys and adrenals as well as cultivating a strong and supple spine. This pose works the postural muscles of the back to improve the posture and therefore the health of the spine and nervous system as well.

Locust Pose (stay for 5–10 breaths, 2–3 times)

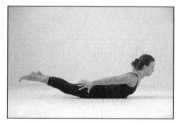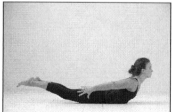

Roll shoulders back, lift sternum, lift inner thighs, reach out through top of head and tips of toes, unclench glutes.

10: Boat Pose (Week Two): Repeat 3-5 rounds, 5 breaths each

11: Bridge Pose (Week Two): Repeat 3-5 rounds, 5-10 breaths each

12: Shoulder Stand (*Sarvangasana*)

Shoulder stand is a very important inversion when done properly. As I stated previously, this book is not meant to be a substitute for yoga instruction so if you haven't done this pose before I recommend learning it under a teacher's guidance. The benefits of this pose could go on for pages and would cover just about every organ and system of the body. For our purposes this pose is important in detoxification for its inverted effects of bringing the blood back to the heart. The veins bring blood back to the heart; unlike the arteries, they rely on valves and the muscle contractions around them to push the blood through them back to the heart. The inversions encourage the return of blood through gravity to take out toxins and revitalize the blood.

Shoulder Stand (hold for 1–4 minutes or 10–20 breaths)

Reach up through feet, legs press into each other, shoulders roll back out of ears and shoulder blades draw together so that none of the vertebra press into the floor, chin away from the chest so there is a natural curve in the neck.

Option: If this is too much on the neck, use a blanket under the shoulders to lift the head and neck off the floor or lay with your legs up the wall and hips on the floor or skip the pose.

13: Fish Pose (*Matsyasana*)

This pose stimulates both the kidneys and adrenals as well as expanding the chest and benefiting the lungs. Traditionally it is used as a counter pose to shoulderstand as well.

Fish Pose (5-10 breaths)

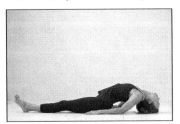

Press through elbows to lift the chest, press sitting bones down to lift low back away from the floor, top of the head is light on the floor, elbows and shoulders away from the ears.

14: Twist (Week Two): Hold for 5-10 breaths each side

15: Pigeon Pose (*Eka Pada Rajakpotasana*)

Pigeon Pose is an important pose for the hips and lower back. Many people carry tension, physical and emotional, in this area making it an important pose to come back to. Tension in this area often contributes to hip and lower back pain and stiffness. There are several layers of muscles in the area so depending where you are tight will determine where you will feel it. The beauty of this pose is that as you start to release some of the superficial muscles you can get into some of the deeper musculature of the hip with the same pose.

Pigeon Pose (1–2 minutes on each side)

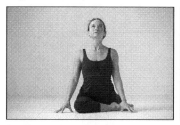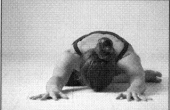
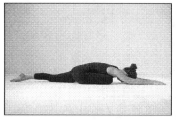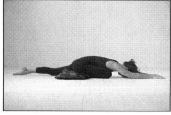

Find a place you can relax into and get a nice hip stretch, keep the foot in close to you for an easier stretch (you should never feel discomfort in the knee in this pose).

Option: If hip is off the floor, put a block or rolled blanket under it (lower right photo) so you can relax; there shouldn't be any discomfort in the knee.

16: Savasana (Week One): 3-5 minutes

Take Savasana for 3-5 minutes, then come to a comfortable seated position on a cushion or rolled blanket for meditation.

17: Meditation with Mindfulness

Mindfulness meditation is a technique that focuses your awareness so it can tap right into your relaxation response. When you sit to meditate, pay attention to the sensation at the tip of the nose with every inhalation and exhalation. Start by observing your whole nose; as you get more practiced in this meditation, you can narrow your focus to the end of the nostrils and then to the space between the upper lip and the nose. Eventually you can concentrate on an area the size of the tip of a pin.

ॐ **Yoga Index**
For a complete rundown of all poses in this program, please see the Yoga Index.

Day Fifteen

Today, as you start Week Two, think about and plan for the coming days.

- Read the section on carbohydrates in the Nutrition chapter.
- Write down your exercise goals for this week.
- Plan time for a sauna this week.
- Continue your daily yoga practice and the weekly overview tasks.

Here's the breakdown:

Carbohydrate Education. Read the Carbohydrates section in the Nutrition chapter and start to incorporate this information into your daily eating.

Activity Goals. Take time today to write down your specific exercise goals for this week.

Sweat It Out. Find time this week to sweat. Many spas or clubs will let you use their sauna for a small fee. Call around and find a way to sweat out some of those toxins this week. Try to sweat vigorously 2-5 times this week (make sure you replace your electrolytes and water afterwards). A hot yoga class will help you sweat, but take some time to relax in a sauna one day instead of hot yoga if that is what you normally do. If you are used to doing Bikram yoga, you may want to try some unheated classes and take some time to relax in a sauna instead. Due to the fact that you lose vital minerals when you sweat I don't recommend doing both.

Dietary Changes. Drink the cranberry beverage. Continue decreasing sugar, alcohol, caffeine, wheat and dairy.

Yoga Practice. Follow the yoga sequence described in the Week Three overview.

Day Sixteen

Small things—like flowers—can change your attitude about the day.

- Buy some flowers for your house or office.
- Explore some more myofascial release.
- Continue your daily yoga practice and the weekly overview tasks.

Here's the breakdown:

Flower Day. Keep it simple today. Make this your motto for the day:

don't over think or overextend yourself. Buy some flowers today to re-mind yourself of your dedication to a better life!

Dietary Changes. Drink the cranberry beverage. Continue decreasing sugar, alcohol, caffeine, wheat and dairy.

Yoga Practice. Follow the yoga sequence described in the Week Three overview.

Myofascial Release. Explore some new, possibly overlooked areas of you body today as we add in some techniques to release the hips and thighs.

Hip Release

These are great techniques for releasing the gluts and hip rotators that are tight and often the culprit of low back pain, knee injuries and poor ankle biomechanics. This one takes some playing with to learn how to leverage the body weight to get deeper into the hips but extremely powerful when used properly. You must be able to relax here; do not clench or grip and think you're helping yourself because it's more painful that way. Part of exercise is to retrain the muscles to learn how to relax properly so that they can also contract more efficiently when they need to.

For this one you will need two tennis balls. Refer to these photos for proper placement of the tennis balls.

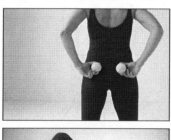
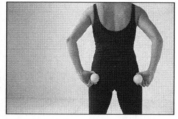
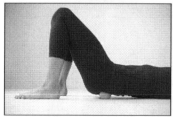
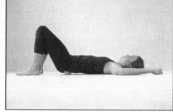

Lie on your back with your knees bent and your feet on the floor. Lift the hips and place the tennis balls on each side of the top of the sacrum just off the bone. Relax completely for 1-2 minutes using the weight of the body to relax the muscles, then move the balls down a few inches at a time and repeat. Next bring the balls back to where you started and move the balls 2-3 inches wider and relax, moving down a few inches at a time stopping at the tender or tight areas for at least a minute or two.

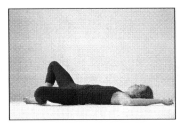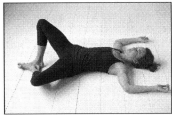

As you get better at knowing your hips and your tight spots, play with moving the leg out to the side so the knee comes out to the side toward the floor, then maybe do both legs together as well as rolling onto one side at a time.

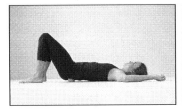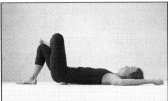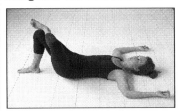

Lie on your back and bend your knees to place your feet on the floor. Make sure you have some room to move around here. Lift the hips and place the tennis balls on either side of the sacrum about 3–4 inches off the bone. Take your right ankle and place it on your left knee so that the right knee moves away from you. Flex your right foot. Place both feet back on the floor and then move the balls wider or lower until you find a tender or tight spot and repeat, relaxing into the tender areas for at least 1–2 minutes then repeat on the other side. When you get better at this one you can do the same thing with the knees bent, feet together and lifting the feet off the floor so that the weight rests over the hips on the tennis balls.

Thigh, Knee and Hip Release

This is great for most knee pain; also for pain in the front of the hip, IT-band syndrome or preventively for runners, cyclists, soccer, tennis, football or any sport that involves a lot of running or side to side movement.

For this one you will need a foam roller or a tennis ball. Refer to photos for placement of tennis balls.

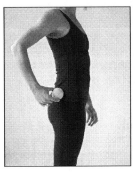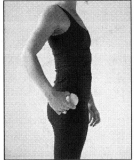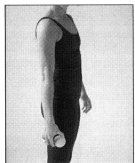

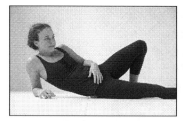 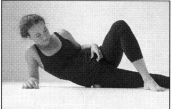

Start by lying on one side with the roller or tennis ball under the hip, supporting yourself on your forearm and rolling down until you find a tender area.
Stop to relax for a minute, then continue all the way down the side of the leg
until you get to the knee.

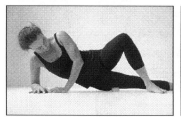 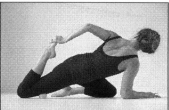

Repeat, this time rolling forward so that you're somewhere between the side
of the leg and the front of the leg, and then repeat lying on the stomach to
get the front of the thigh. For the front of the thigh, if you're happy there, find
a tight spot and then prop up on the forearm and bend the knee to reach
back and grab the ankle for a deeper release.

Dietary Changes. Drink the cranberry beverage. Continue decreasing
sugar, alcohol, caffeine, wheat and dairy.

Yoga Practice. Follow the yoga sequence described in the Week Three
overview.

Day Seventeen

Because Week Three targets the skin, today try these techniques to make
your skin glow.

- Do hydrotherapy or dry skin brushing.
- Try myofascial release on your neck.
- Continue your daily yoga practice and the weekly overview tasks.

Here's the breakdown:

Skin Refresh. Take time today to use some simple hydrotherapy or dry
skin brushing to aid the detoxification process. Below are some simple
options you can do yourself at home.

- **Hydrotherapy.** Water is an excellent temperature medium. It can retain cold and heat in a form that can easily be applied to the body. These temperatures help to aid in the dilation (heat) and constriction (cold) of blood vessels. This change in the blood vessels allows for improved circulation, better waste removal and faster healing. I'm a huge fan of hydrotherapy; here are a few of my favorites:

  - *Therapeutic Contrast Shower.* After you shower, turn down the temperature of the hot water as low as you can tolerate (eventually you may be able to completely turn down the hot water). Cover every inch of your body with the cool water, including the bottoms of your feet. Focus the cold stream on any achy or painful areas: back, joints, pelvis, etc. Then alternate hot and cold and end with a little cold. Do the cold for about 30 seconds and the hot water for about 1 minute, just long enough for your body to adapt to the new temperature. Repeat 1-3 times, then dry yourself off quickly, rubbing briskly. It is important to feel very warm internally before beginning the cold phase. For a daily hydrotherapy treatment, finish your hot morning shower with a blast of cold water.

    This therapy helps strengthen and normalize the nervous, circulatory, endocrine (hormonal), musculoskeletal and immune systems, and is excellent for helping the body cope with stress. Alternating between hot and cold stimulates blood circulation and lymphatic flow. The more you challenge yourself with cold, the more you will notice these effects, sometimes even a subtle healthy high. There may be times when you feel more sensitive to the cold; in this case you should either temporarily decrease the intensity or discontinue this treatment.

  - *Constitutional Hydrotherapy.* Perhaps the most powerful and useful of all water treatments, constitutional hydrotherapy is a special technique that can greatly improve recovery from a wide variety of acute and chronic illnesses. This treatment is helpful in any case where detoxification, immune stimulation and digestion enhancement are needed. Take a hot shower for at least five minutes. Get out and dry quickly. Take a towel wrung out in cold water and wrap it around the trunk of the body, from armpit to groin. Cover entire body with a large wool blanket. Leave cold towel in place for at least 20 minutes, or longer, until the towel is warmed up.

- *Cold/Flu Fighter.* After taking a warm shower, rinse a small, thin piece of cotton (handkerchief or bandana) in cold water and ring out thoroughly, then wrap around the neck. Cover the cloth and the entire neck with a wool cloth/scarf, go straight to bed and do not remove until the morning (the cloth will be dry when you wake up). Sleep overnight with this on. It sounds uncomfortable but it feels great and will kick out even the worst of cold or flu if you catch it early. It's simple and easy. I love to use this one if I feel like I'm just starting to get a sore throat or swollen glands.

- *Salt Glow.* The salt glow, in which the body is rubbed vigorously with sea salts or Epsom salts, is an invigorating treatment for those with poor circulation. It's also recommended as preventive medicine or for those following a detoxification program. Starting with damp skin, take a handful of moistened sea salts or Epsom salts and massage your skin vigorously until it turns slightly pink. Repeat on the arms, legs, back, shoulders and abdomen—and don't forget the hands and feet. The salt glow may make you perspire but it will help you sleep more soundly.

- *Seaweed Detox Bath.* For a powerful detoxifying bath, use mineral-rich seaweed and Epsom salt. Sea salt is purifying and baking soda softens the skin for a smooth feel. Here's the recipe:

  - 1 cup Epsom salt
  - ½ cup dried kelp or dulse
  - ½ cup sea salt:
  - 1 cup baking soda

  Grind the seaweed into a powder by hand or in a blender. Add the entire mix to your warm or hot bath. Soak for 20 minutes and rinse with cold water.

- **Wet Socks.** This is a simple but powerful remedy. Most people who experience poor-quality sleep report that their sleep quickly improves with this wet sock treatment. It's an old folk remedy, tested and true. It's great for colds, sinus infections, sore throats, ear infections, coughs, insomnia and much more. Great for kids, too. Surprisingly, they typically don't complain about having cold wet socks put on their feet. Here's what to do:

Tip: Salt on your Skin Don't use salt rubs if you have a rash or sensitive skin.

- Supplies:
    - 1 pair white cotton socks
    - 1 pair thick wool socks (as close to 100% wool as possible)
- Directions:

    1. Wet cotton socks and soak them completely with cold water. Be sure to wring the socks out thoroughly so they do not drip. If you desire, place wet socks in the freezer for 3–5 minutes (do not freeze if using this treatment on children).

    2. While cotton socks are chilling, warm your feet. This is very important to increase the efficacy of the treatment. Warming can be accomplished by soaking your feet in warm water for at least 5-10 minutes or taking a warm shower or bath.

    3. Dry the feet off completely.

    4. Place cold wet socks on feet. Cover with thick wool socks. Go directly to bed. Avoid getting chilled.

    5. Keep the socks on overnight. The cotton socks should be dry in the morning.

This treatment works by forcing the circulation down through the legs at night to dry the socks from the inside. The increased circulation supports drainage in the sinuses and throat while you sleep. Typically during the night our circulation throughout the body is very stagnant. This treatment changes that dynamic.

Please *do not* remove socks in the middle of the night. This is a common mistake and will ruin the effectiveness of the treatment. They may still be wet in the middle of the night, but trust that they will be dry in the morning. Many patients also report that they sleep much better during the treatment.

- **Dry-Skin Brushing.** This technique helps rid the skin of toxins and dead cells. It also helps with blood and lymphatic circulation as well as cellulite. It does require a special dry skin brush that you can buy at Whole Foods or your local natural grocery store. Starting at the feet use circular strokes to brush back toward the heart, do the whole body except the face, genitals and any areas with acne, eczema, psoriasis or cuts.

Myofascial Release. Continue myofascial techniques to release the neck and base of the skull.

Neck and Occiput Release

This one is phenomenal for headaches, migraines, cervical range of motion, sinus congestion and eye pain or strain from the computer.

You will need a foam roller or yoga block—I prefer a block for more integrity.

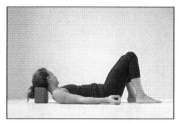

Lie on your back with the base of the skull on your foam roller or the edge of your block and completely relax the neck so that the head is heavy. Slowly roll the head side to side and look for tender or tight areas. Stopping at tight spots for a minute or two to inhale into this area and exhaling to relax the muscles.

Dietary Changes. Drink the cranberry beverage. Continue decreasing sugar, alcohol, caffeine, wheat and dairy.

Yoga Practice. Follow the yoga sequence described in the Week Three overview.

Day Eighteen

As you deepen your awareness of your body through yoga, it's important to see how yoga connects to your approach to life.

- ♦ Go on a television fast.

- ♦ Study yoga philosophy.

- ♦ Continue your daily yoga practice and the weekly overview tasks.

Here's the breakdown:

Television Fast. Abstain from television again today. Use this time to read about the traditional yogic philosophy and to cultivate some inner silence.

Yoga Philosophy. Although there are many styles of yoga, there is one thing that all styles of yoga agree on and that's the Eight Limbs of Yoga, the essence upon which all practices are based. Today you'll explore the first four limbs, which are all very relevant and applicable to our daily lives. Write in your journal again today. Take some notes on what these limbs of yoga mean to you.

☜Thought: Minute by Minute
Continue your one positive attribute. Begin each day with it, even if just for a minute.

ॐ *The Eight Limbs of Yoga*

1. **Yamas** *(don'ts)*
2. **Niyamas** *(do's)*
3. **Asana**
4. **Pranayama** *(breath/energy control)*
5. **Pratyahara** *(withdrawal of the senses)*
6. **Dharana** *(one-pointed focus)*
7. **Dhyana** *(meditation, sustained focus or absorption)*
8. **Samadhi** *(enlightenment)*

Let's look at these first four more closely.

1. **Yamas** *(Moral Restrictions)*

   ♦ *Ahimsa*

   - Non-violence
   - Never to harm or demean
   - Compassion
   - Never to wish harm in any way, non-judging
   - Upon mastery it is said that all creatures become harmless in your presence

   ♦ *Satya*

   - Non-lying, truthfulness
   - Never say what isn't so with intent to deceive
   - Be genuine and authentic
   - Truthfulness must be practiced with non-violence, it must come from love
   - Self honesty
   - Before speaking always contemplate: is it truthful, is it necessary, is it the appropriate time and can it be said in a kind way?
   - Upon mastery it is said that whatever one says will come true

   ♦ *Asteya*

   - Non-stealing
   - Not taking what isn't yours, material or not (credit for actions)

- Not desire what isn't yours, even praise, status, time or love
- Don't build yourself up at another's expense
- See everything as a part of yourself
- Letting go of ownership
- Upon mastery it is said that whatever you need comes to you when you need it

- ◆ *Brahmacharya*

  - Moderation in all things
  - Control of the senses, not overindulging in the senses
  - What is it your body is really craving?
  - Directing one's sexual energy with integrity
  - Learning to enjoy the good in everything
  - Upon mastery it is said that one gains mental clarity and good health on all levels

- ◆ *Aparigraha*

  - Non-greed
  - Non-hoarding, non-possessiveness
  - Letting go of attachments, even things that are yours by right
  - It is OK to have things; this is more about your attachment to those things

2. **Niyamas** (*Moral Practices*)

- ◆ *Saucha*

  - Cleanliness
  - Orderliness, precision
  - Purity of body and environment, as well as in deed and thought
  - Upon mastery one will find indifference to things of the body

- ◆ *Santosha*

  - Contentment
  - The ability to embrace things as they are
  - Accepting what is
  - Equanimity
  - Being present, the present is the only moment we truly have
  - Upon mastery one finds unceasing inner happiness and bliss

ॐ **The Eight Limbs of Yoga**
Based on the writings of Patanjali, generally considered to the founder of what we know as yoga today, the Eight Limbs of Ashtanga yoga form the essence of Raja yoga, which incorporates meditation into its practice.

- *Tapas*
  - Self discipline, simplicity, removal of distraction
  - This discipline is the fire that one goes through in life, like refining gold
  - Seeing suffering as an opportunity for change
  - Mastery over likes and dislikes
- *Swadhyaya*
  - Self study
  - Mindfulness
  - Introspection of one's behavior, motives, desires, etc
  - Reflection
- *Ishvarapranidhana*
  - Surrender
  - To let go of the ego

3. **Asana**

We're all familiar with this one: this practice is meant to purify and calm the body and mind to prepare for meditation.

4. **Pranayama**

- *Breath control, also energy control*
- *Using the breath to regulate the body, mind and nervous system*

Dietary Changes. Drink the cranberry beverage. Continue decreasing sugar, alcohol, caffeine, wheat and dairy.

Yoga Practice. Follow the yoga sequence described in the Week Three overview.

Day Nineteen

Today plan to experience other regenerative treatments. Question your attachment to unhealthy kitchen utensils as well.

- Schedule acupuncture or massage this week or next.
- Take stock of plastics and microwaves.
- Try using a neti pot.
- Continue your daily yoga practice and the weekly overview tasks.

Here's the breakdown:

Acupuncture and Massage. Acupuncture and massage have many different uses that can be used as prevention or as treatment for specific issues. Below are some of the ways each of these is used for preventative wellness.

Acupuncture can:

- Regulate energy fluctuations
- Stimulate the immune system
- Repair/regulate musculoskeletal system
- Regulate thyroid and adrenal function
- Regulate digestion and absorption
- Act as an anti-inflammatory for pain or indigestion
- Regulate the nervous system and hormone levels/cycles
- Stimulate detoxification
- Help regulate the metabolism and cravings
- Stimulate the body's own healing mechanism
- Be used for general maintenance

Massage can:

- Encourage lymphatic drainage and circulation to aid detoxification
- Allow relaxation-mentally and physically
- Help repair or maintain muscle/tendon elasticity
- Be used for general maintenance

Plastics and Microwaves. Plastics, especially when heated, release harmful chemicals that can interfere with your body's hormones (estrogen, thyroid, etc.). Microwaves can disrupt chemical bonds in otherwise healthy foods, decreasing the nutritional content. Start minimizing your use of plastics, microwaves and Teflon/non-stick pans—use stainless steel instead.

Neti Pot (*Jala Neti*). Neti pot or nasal irrigation is an ancient Indian cleansing technique known as Jala neti, which literally means "cleansing with water" in Sanskrit. It's a common practice in parts of India and Southeast Asia that's used routinely, like brushing your teeth. Usually

☯ **Thought: Gratefully Alive**
As you approach your yoga practice today, make it an act of appreciation for your body and your health. For every breath we take we should be grateful that we are still here walking, living and breathing!

performed daily first thing in the morning and maybe at the end of the day as well, it can be used up to four times a day for more serious sinus issues. Jala neti is especially helpful for people who work or live in polluted environments or suffer from sinus infections or more chronic sinus problems.

- **What it does:** Jala neti rinses out the dirt- and bacteria-filled mucous lining of the sinuses. The warm water loosens and dissolves any internal build up and the sinus passages are drained by the vacuum pressure of the flow of water. For many people the relief can be felt within seconds. Neti is more traditionally used as a pre-requisite for cleaning the respiratory passages prior to pranayama practice. According to yoga philosophy, balancing the nasal breathing function results in better balance of the sympathetic and parasympathetic nervous systems and hence better balance of the entire nervous system. Therefore, one of the uses in yogic philosophy is to relieve mental tension and headaches. Here are some other uses:

  - Clear out mucus and reduce nasal congestion

  - Cleanse and rid the sinus cavities of allergens and irritants

  - Helps with chronic sinusitis, acute sinus infections and allergic rhinitis

  - Relieve nasal dryness

  - Promote healthy nasal passages and improve breathing

- **How to use it:** The goal is to reduce or eliminate recurrent irritants so that the body can be given a chance to heal itself. Long-term use of the neti pot along with appropriate diet and lifestyle changes can be extremely helpful for the conditions mentioned above. It is important to follow the instructions carefully. Continue using as maintenance or until symptoms resolve, which may take up to three to six months, so be patient. For acute problems, repeat up to four times per day until resolved. For chronic problems, it is useful to do the wash one or more times daily, continuing for several months. Be persistent: it takes a lot of effort to rid your body of chronic irritants and bacteria. If your symptoms continue to worsen or no improvement is noted after a week of treatment, consult your healthcare practitioner.

Jala Neti Supplies:

> ½ tsp unrefined sea salt (pure sea salt should have small gray specks in it)

1 cup filtered or distilled water

Neti pot

Paper towels and tissues

Directions:

1. Fill the neti pot with salt and warm water (as warm as you can tolerate). The salt-to-water ratio is ½ teaspoon sea salt to 1 cup water. Filtered water is best.

2. Have some tissues within reach for this next part. Over a sink, tilt your head forward so that you are looking directly down toward the sink. Insert the spout into your right nostril. It's important that you relax and breathe through your mouth. Turn your head to the left and let the water move into the right nostril and exit the left nostril. Normally, you will feel the water as it passes through your sinuses. It's fine if some of the water drains into the mouth, simply spit it out and adjust the tilt of your head further forward so that all or most of the water comes out the opposite nostril.

3. After using half of the mixture, repeat the above procedure for the other nostril.

4. To finish, gently expel the water by bending forward with a towel over your face and your nose pointing toward the floor. Gently blow air out both open nostrils several times, then stand upright and repeating this. Avoid the temptation to block off one nostril, as doing so may force water into the Eustachian tubes. Once the passages are mostly dry you may gently blow the nose as needed.

• **Common Problems.** If there are hardened blockages or you are unable to get the water to go through the sinuses, apply a warm compress with a little eucalyptus oil for a few minutes to open the sinuses enough to get water through. Hardened blockages will loosen slowly over time. If there is burning or irritation, make sure the salt level is correct and that you are using filtered water. If it still persists, try distilled water or warmer or cooler water. The sensitivity should decrease over time when done correctly. If you experience discomfort in your ear, make sure you are gently blowing the nose afterwards. Discontinue if you have sharp or persistent problems or pain.

Dietary Changes. Drink the cranberry beverage. Continue decreasing sugar, alcohol, caffeine, wheat and dairy.

Yoga Practice. Follow the yoga sequence described in the Week Three overview.

Day Twenty

Your feet not only transport you, but they ground you as well. Today, give them the attention they deserve.

- Enjoy a detoxifying footbath.

- Practice more myofascial release.

- Continue your daily yoga practice and the weekly overview tasks.

Here's the breakdown:

Foot Detoxification. Try a detoxifying footbath before bed. The footbath in itself will help calm the nervous system to prepare you for a deeper, more restful sleep. Here are some types of treatments to choose from:

- Epsom salts: detoxifying and relaxing (¼ cup)

- Baking soda: alkalinizing, good for skin irritations (2 oz.)

- Seaweed: detoxifies and re-mineralizes (½-1 oz., powdered or micronized)

- Essential oils: Juniper berry, rosemary or grapefruit are all detoxifying (use 2-6 drops)

Myofascial Release. Continue myofascial techniques to release the feet and back.

Foot Release

The feet do so much for us and are often a source of tension from walking, running, poorly fitting shoes, pointed toes or heels. The fascia on the back side of the body begins on the underside of the foot and continues up the back of the calves, hamstrings, sacrum, low mid- and upper-back and neck to the back of the skull. Because of the fascial tension contribution this release can help any of these areas.

For this one you will need a tennis ball or golf ball.

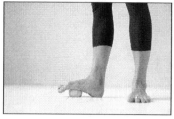 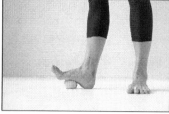 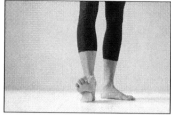

Stand or sit with your foot on the tennis ball. Gently roll out the underside of the foot. Obviously this will be more intense with more pressure on the foot, but you can also use a golf ball to intensify it or play with curling and extending the toes as you do it.

Back Release

This is a great technique for releasing the tight erector spinae muscles along the sides of the spine that are often overused and strained in many cases of lower back pain. This can also be a very calming technique for the nervous system to counteract stress or to help you relax before bed.

You will need two tennis balls. Refer to the photo for proper placement of the tennis balls.

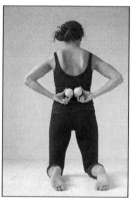 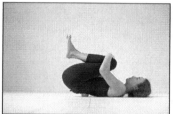 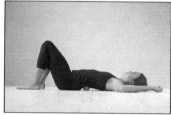

Lie on your back and put your calves up on a chair or couch so that the knees are over the hips and the hips are on the floor, or with knees bent and feet on the floor. Lift the hips and place the tennis balls on either side of the spine around the mid spine area. Start with the tennis balls close together so that they touch and relax completely for 1–2 minutes using the weight of the body to relax the muscles. Then move the balls down a few inches and repeat going all the way down the spine and sacrum, stopping at the tender or tight areas for at least a couple minutes. As you get better at knowing your back and your tight spots you can go right to the tight areas or play with moving the balls wider apart. You can also move the balls up along the spine for mid or upper back tension, playing with the width of the balls as well to focus into the tightest areas.

Dietary Changes. Drink the cranberry beverage. Continue decreasing sugar, alcohol, caffeine, wheat and dairy.

Yoga Practice. Follow the yoga sequence described in the Week Three overview.

Tip: Many of the supplements mentioned in this book are available at *www.TiffanyYoga.com.*

Day Twenty-One

Today explore herbal supplements that can rejuvenate and restore your body and mind. Plus, prepare for your final week.

- Learn about adaptogenic herbs.

- Buy supplies for next week.

- Continue your daily yoga practice and the weekly overview tasks.

Here's the breakdown:

Adaptogenic Herbs. Today we are going to look at how a group of herbs called the adaptogens can affect your health. The term adaptogen is used by herbalists to refer to an herb that increases the body's resistance to stress, trauma, anxiety and fatigue. In the past, they have been called rejuvenating herbs, tonics or restoratives. All adaptogens contain antioxidants, but antioxidants are not necessarily adaptogens—it's not their primary mode of action. Here's what they do:

- An adaptogen produces a nonspecific response in the body—an increased resistance to multiple stressors including physical, chemical or biological agents.

- An adaptogen has a normalizing influence on physiology, capable of either toning down the activity of hyperfunctioning systems or strengthening the activity of hypofunctioning systems.

There are many really great adaptogens that are coming to the market and are getting a lot of press. Choose one or two from this list or discover your own favorites or find a supplement at your local health food store that contains several of these herbs. Most stores sell at least one or two (sometimes they are listed as tonics or adrenal tonics or for stress, etc.) Follow the dose listed on the bottle. Generally adaptogens are taken between meals to maximize absorption; however, if it bothers your stomach, take it with a little food. Here are a few of my favorites.

- **Eleuthero**, also known as Siberian Ginseng, is a distant relative of American *Panax quinquefolius*) and Asian ginseng (*Panax ginseng*). But it's a distinct plant with different active chemical components. Prized for its ability to restore vigor, increase longevity, enhance overall health and stimulate both a healthy appetite and a good memory, it's widely used in Russia to help the body adapt to stressful conditions and to enhance productivity. In Chinese medicine, it is valued for its beneficial effects on *qi* and its ability to treat *yang* deficiency in the spleen and kidney (fatigue, unmotivated, tend to be cold, indigestion, etc).

The active ingredients in Siberian ginseng, called eleutherosides, are thought to increase stamina and to stimulate the immune system. Siberian ginseng may help the body deal with physically and mentally stressful exposures, such as heat, cold, physical exhaustion, viruses, bacteria, chemicals, extreme working conditions, noise and pollution. (Take 500 mg of Eleuthero 3 times/day between meals if taken alone, use less if mixed with other herbs.)

- **Astragalus** (*Astragalus membranaceus*) has been used in traditional Chinese medicine for thousands of years, often in combination with other herbs, to strengthen the body's resistance to disease. It contains antioxidants that protect cells against damage caused by free radicals, which are by-products of cellular energy. Astragalus is well known for its ability to protect and support the immune system, for preventing colds and upper respiratory infections, to lower blood pressure, treat diabetes and protect the liver.

Astragalus has antibacterial, anti-inflammatory and diuretic properties. Studies have shown that astragalus has antiviral properties and stimulates the immune system, suggesting that it is indeed effective at preventing colds. In the United States, researchers have investigated astragalus as a possible treatment for people whose immune systems have been compromised by chemotherapy or radiation. In these studies, astragalus supplements have been shown to speed recovery and extend life expectancy.

- **Ashwagandha**, also known as Indian Winter Cherry, is a shrub cultivated in India and North America whose roots have been used for thousands of years by Ayurvedic practitioners. Several studies over the past few years have examined ashwagandha's anti-inflammatory, anti-tumor, anti-stress, antioxidant, mind-boosting, immune-enhancing and rejuvenating properties. Historically ashwagandha root has also been noted to enhance the libido and sexual functions as well.

The latest research has revealed that ashwagandha can restore neurotransmitters for various mental disorders and can be useful to calm the mind and promote sound, restful sleep. As with all the adaptogens, ashwagandha is helpful for any stress-related disorders.

Thought: Notice how much your expectations affect your day. What you expect from the day can affect its outcome. Your perception can help you decide how you approach life.

- **Holy Basil** (*Ocimum sanctum*) is an herb native to India, where it is known as *tulsi*. It is sacred in the Hindu religious tradition and is regarded as one of the most important plants used in Ayurvedic medicine. If you go to India, you will see holy basil growing in profusion around Hindu temples. It comes in red and green varieties, both with a strong, pleasant aroma.

  In the past decade or so a number of scientific studies have looked at holy basil for various treatment purposes. Findings from these various investigations suggest that holy basil might have some effects as a painkiller, a COX-II anti-inflammatory agent, an antioxidant and as a treatment for bacterial, fungal and even viral infections. There is also evidence that holy basil can help control blood sugar. Holy basil is well known to help counteract the effects of stress; preparations made from holy basil are widely used to treat stress-related health problems in India and elsewhere.

- **Rhodiola** (*Rhodiola rosea*), sometimes called Arctic root or golden root, grows at high altitudes in the arctic areas of Europe and Asia, and its root has been used in traditional medicine in Russia and the Scandinavian countries for centuries. Studies of its medicinal applications have appeared in the scientific literature of Sweden, Norway, France, Germany, the Soviet Union and Iceland. Today rhodiola is used as a tonic and remedy for fatigue, poor attention span, mild depression and decreased memory.

  A 2002 review in *Herbalgram, The Journal of the American Botanical Council*, reported that over the years, numerous studies of rhodiola in humans and animals have shown that it helps prevent fatigue, stress and the damaging effects of oxygen deprivation. Evidence also suggests that it has an antioxidant effect, enhances immune system function and can increase sexual energy. A study published in 2007 in the *Nordic Journal of Psychiatry* showed that patients with mild-to-moderate depression who took a rhodiola extract reported fewer symptoms than those who took a placebo. And a study by researchers at the University of California at Irvine found that fruit flies that ate a diet supplemented with rhodiola lived an average of 10 percent longer than flies that didn't eat this herb.

These are a few of my favorites, but there are so many more adaptogenic herbs to choose from. You can also check out Reishi, Maca and Cordyceps.

Go Shopping. Buy supplies for next week:

- Sole supplies: Pink Himalayan Sea Salt (Week Four)
- Adaptogenic herbs (Day 21)
- Probiotics (Week Four)

Dietary Changes. Drink the cranberry beverage. Continue decreasing sugar, alcohol, caffeine, wheat and dairy.

Yoga Practice. Follow the yoga sequence described in the Week Three overview.

Congratulations! You're entering the home stretch of your optimal health and detoxification program.

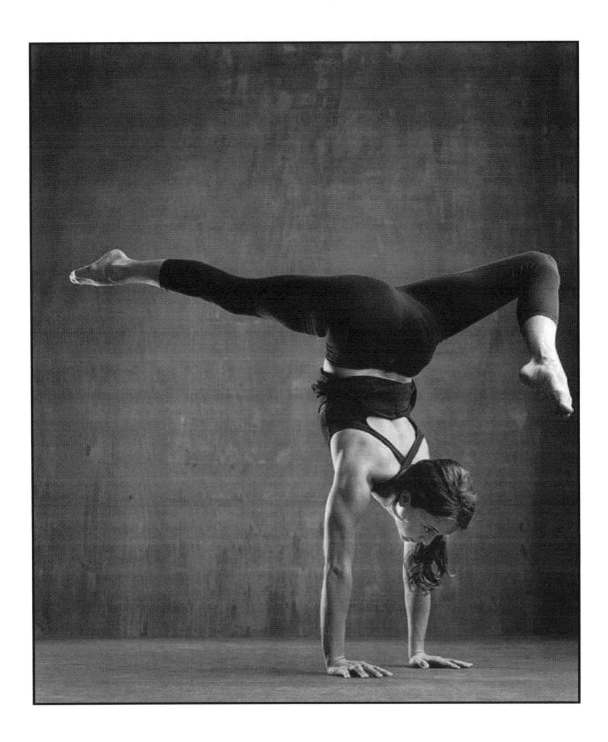

Week Four

Everything that you say to yourself or believe about yourself
affects you mentally, physically and emotionally.
Thinking positively can greatly change your outlook
and reduce your stress levels.

— page 130

Week Four: Restore and Revitalize

In this final week of the Optimal Health Program, we focus on nourishing the body and strengthening the adrenal and immune systems. Over time stress weakens our system and makes it more susceptible to toxins. Now that you have thoroughly cleansed your body, this week you'll strengthen your resilience to disease.

Week Four is about moderation. You will still limit these foods for the most part—sugar, alcohol, caffeine, wheat and dairy—but not necessarily completely eliminate them. However, moderation can be difficult, especially in our all-or-nothing society.

Here is what you'll be doing all week long:

rock-at Whole Foods

1. Drink sole.

2. Take adaptogenic herbs and probiotics.

3. Limit sugar, alcohol, caffeine, wheat and dairy.

4. Continue your daily yoga and meditation practice this week.

As with the previous weeks, fill out an overview chart to set your goals for the week:

Sole	
Adaptogenic herbs	
Probiotics	
Sugar/alcohol/ caffeine	
Dairy/wheat	
Yoga	

Let's take a closer look at each of these.

Drink Sole. The ancient Celts believed that all life originated in the ocean, the "sole" of the sea. In German, the word "sole," is derived from the Latin word "sol," which means sun. Sole is a drink made from pink Himalayan salt and is said to be the fluid materialization of sunlight. When water combines with salt, the positive ions of the salt surround the negative ions of the water molecules, and the negative ions of the salt surround the positive ions of the water molecules so that the ions become hydrolyzed. In this

📖 **FYI: Pink Himalayan Salt**
Much purer than sea salt, this marine fossil salt harvested from the foothills of the Himalayas, is 100 percent natural, unrefined and unpolluted. Pink Himalayan salt combines the incredible flavor from the ancient sea with rich minerals including calcium, magnesium, potassium, copper and iron. This salt has the same mineral profile as human blood and is therefore very nourishing to the body unlike refined salt that can actually leach minerals from the body.

process the geometrical structure of the salt and the water is changed and a new structure is formed.

Sole supplies the body with the natural energy stored in the salt crystals to:

- Harmonize alkalinity/acidity
- Re-mineralize the body
- Regulate blood pressure
- Dissolve and eliminate sediments that lead to stones and various forms of rheumatism, like arthritis and kidney and gall bladder stones
- Increase circulation through the body and oxygenation of the cells
- Help with skin diseases by cleansing from inside out
- Balance the pH and eliminate heavy metals
- Helps balance the endocrine system

- **Making Sole.** Place 1–2 rocks of pink Himalayan salt in a glass jar with filtered water and cover, completely covering the crystals with water and let sit overnight.

If all the salt crystals have dissolved, add more salt to the water. Your Himalayan sole is ready when the water becomes fully saturated with salt and cannot hold any more. There should always be salt crystals at the bottom of the jar. As you use up the sole, add more water and more salt until the water is again saturated. Remember, there should always be undissolved salt crystals on the bottom of the jar. This is your visual proof that the water is totally saturated with salt.

It is estimated that one teaspoon of Sole contains approximately .01 gram of salt. At that concentration it would take 100 teaspoons of Sole to make 1 gram of salt so there is no need to worry about overdosing. Our society has grown to fear salt but when you add salt that nourishes the body versus one that is toxic the outcome is quite different. Salt is a core essential nutrient with exceptional qualities fundamental for keeping us alive and healthy.

Pink Himalayan salt can often be found at smaller cooperative natural grocery stores or you can find it at several websites online.

Each morning, before eating or drinking anything, take one teaspoon of sole in or with a large glass of filtered water.

Take Adaptogenic Herbs. This week, start taking the adaptogenic herbs that you chose on Day 21.

Take Probiotics. Probiotics are a one of the best things you can do for preventive care of your health. Probiotics are essential for the digestive and immune systems. Research goes on about the many uses for these valuable supplements. Several studies also underscore the importance of probiotics in pregnant women and kids for the development of the immune system for issues like allergies, asthma, skin problems, etc.

When taking probiotics it's important to take a good quality supplement. Consumer Labs tested many of the probiotic brands on the market and found that most lack viable organisms, due to the sensitivity of probiotics to its environment. One that passed the test, and one that I like, is JarrowDophillus by Jarrow. It's relatively easy to find and it's cost friendly. I have my patients take 1 pill once a day for maintenance, or 2 pills two times/day as a therapeutic dose for digestive problems, sinus issues or immune system enhancement. It's best taken first thing in the morning and/or before bed.

Limit sugar, alcohol, caffeine, wheat, dairy and processed foods.
Week Four begins your transition to sustainable eating habits. Because you eliminated sugar and processed food from your diet, you now have a natural internal monitor of your sugar intake and a better idea of the hidden sources of sugar and unhealthy fats in your food. Moderate eating of these foods is key from this point forward, and moderation can be the hardest part.

Some people experience significant changes from eliminating wheat or dairy and may want to cut those out of your diet for a while to eliminate the irritating effects on your system. Others notice the biggest change from getting rid of sugar and alcohol, while still others find biggest effect stems from doing away with caffeine. Whatever you find, key into your biggest return area and maximize the long-term effects by minimizing or eliminating this item(s).

Yoga Practice. This week you will add some more new poses and pranayama and meditation variations. At this point you have plenty of poses to choose from, so feel free to change it up by adding or leaving out some poses. Consider this sequence as a starting point.

If pain or dizziness is experienced, stop the practice and sit quietly for a few minutes. When the sensation has passed, recommence the practice with more awareness and less force. If the problem continues, consult a yoga teacher.

Contra-indications for Kapalabhati: Kapalabhati should not be practiced by those suffering from heart disease, vertigo, epilepsy, stroke, hernia, severe gastric ulcer, recent surgery, emphysema, or during menstruation or pregnancy. Instead do any of the previous pranayama techniques.

Week Four Yoga

This week we add a few more poses to nourish and regulate the adrenal and the immune systems as well as the entire system to make a potent well-rounded practice. Use this as a simple base to add to or subtract from as you like in the future.

1. Kapalabhati Pranayama

Kapalabhati, or kriya, is a breathing technique used specifically for cleansing. Great quantities of carbon dioxide are eliminated during this pranayama. The intake of oxygen makes the blood richer and renews the body tissues. It invigorates the liver, spleen, pancreas, heart, diaphragm and abdominal muscles and improves digestion. It also massages the internal organs, stimulates digestion and elimination, removes stale air and toxins from the lungs, drains the sinuses and pumps fresh prana into the cells of the body. It energizes, massages and cleanses the central nervous system, bringing mental clarity and alertness. This practice also tones the abdominal muscles that support the internal organs to help with core strength and posture. The key to effective Kapalabhati Pranayama, as with all types of pranayama, is to remain relaxed and to stay focused and mindful of what is occurring.

Sit in a comfortable cross-legged position with an erect spine, shoulders wide, sternum lifting with each inhalation. Close your eyes. Take several deep breaths and feel tension leaving the body through each exhalation. Begin with several rounds of deep ujjayi breathing. Then begin Kapalabhati by exhaling forcefully through the nostrils as you contract the abdominal muscles and draw the belly toward the spine. The inhalation happens passively and the belly will relax. Repeat slowly at first to make sure the belly is relaxing after the contraction. Find your rhythm. Remember the emphasis is on the exhalation. You should hear yourself exhale as you force the breath out quickly. Inhalation happens naturally between each exhale without much sound.

Always start slowly, limiting your repetitions until the body is ready to move to the next level. Start with approximately one breath per second with a total of 10-20 breaths per round. At the end of each round exhale completely, then inhale and hold for 5-10 counts. Take 1-3 deep breaths between rounds and do 3 rounds. As you become more comfortable with Kapalabhati, you can increase the repetitions, progressing in 10-15 breath increments, working toward 100 repetitions per round and perhaps two breaths per second. If you feel short of breath slow down to allow more time for the inhalation or stop and lay down. The pumping mechanism should happen deep in the belly not up in the chest like you're hyperventilating.

2: Cat/Cow (Week One): Repeat 5-10 times

3: Tabletop Stability (Week One): Hold for 5-10 breaths each side

4: Sun Salutation, Version A (Week One): Repeat 3-5 times

5: Sun Salutation, Version B (Week One): Repeat 3-5 times

6: Chair Pose and Twist (*Utkatasana* and *Parivritta Utkatasana*)

This pose establishes strength in the gluts, hamstrings, quads and core to create a strong support for the lower back. The revolved variation stimulates the kidneys and adrenals as well as digestion, elimination and liver detoxification.

🌐 **Thought: Nourish the Mind**
As you make our way through this last week, focus on the simple act of nourishing yourself. Make this thought your intention in meditation, yoga, eating, taking your sole and herbs for the day. Adding this simple mindfulness will make these practices much more potent.

Chair Pose (hold for 5–10 breaths)

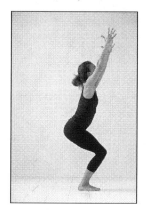

Bases of big toes touch, heels slightly apart, soften shoulders down from ears (left photo).

Chair Pose Twist (5–10 breaths each side)

Lift the heart from between the shoulders, draw the shoulder blades back, knees level with each other (right photo).

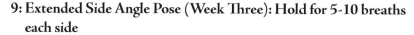

7: Triangle Pose (Week Two): Hold for 5-10 breaths each side

8: Revolved Triangle (Week Two): Hold for 5-10 breaths each side

9: Extended Side Angle Pose (Week Three): Hold for 5-10 breaths each side

10: Half Moon (*Ardha Chandrasana*)

This pose both requires and instills confidence to maintain. It strengthens the lateral support for the lumbar spine which is important for the low back and functional stability and also strengthens the kidneys and adrenals.

Half Moon Pose (5–10 breaths each side)

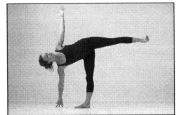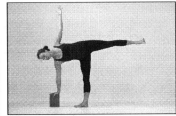

Stack the hips and shoulders, extend through the arms and legs, lift ribs away from pelvis and inflate kidneys to elongate the spine.

Option: Use a block or bend the knee as needed

11: Locust Pose (Week Three): Hold for 5-10 breaths each side

12: Camel Pose (*Utrasana*)

Camel pose is an excellent pose to create strength and suppleness in the spine and nervous system. It is also a tonic for the adrenals and kidneys when done properly and opens the chest to improve the posture and lift some tension off the digestive organs.

Camel Pose (5–10 breaths)

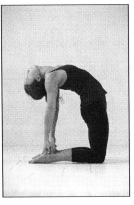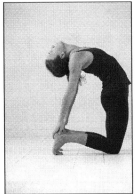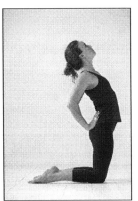

Use the quads to bring you back and keep them active throughout by pressing down through the shins and knees, lift the sternum the entire time with the shoulders rolling back then lift from the sternum with the quads active to lift you up.

Option: Tuck the toes back or just keep the hands on the sacrum for an easier version.

13: Boat Pose (Week Two): Repeat 3-5 rounds, 5 breaths each

14: Bridge Stability

This is a variation on bridge pose that I like for its ability to coordinate pelvic and core stability with the movement of the legs. This is a challenging variation used preventively for the low back and the lower extremities. This pose is better used preventively then during acute lower back pain, if your back is irritated just do bridge with a block between the thighs.

Bridge Stability (5–10 breaths each side)

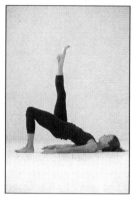 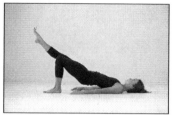

Hips level, press down and out through the feet, scoop belly, reach out through the foot.

15: Bridge Pose (Week Two): Repeat 3-5 rounds, 5-10 breaths each

16: Shoulder Stand (Week Three): Hold for 1-4 minutes or 10-20 breaths

17: Fish Pose (Week Three): Hold 5-10 breaths

18: Headstand (*Shirshasana*): Optional, only if experienced

Headstand is known as "the queen of poses" and is considered to be one of the most important yoga poses. The reason relates to the effect it has on the brain. The inversion aspect of this pose causes increased and unrestricted blood flow to the brain. This brings increased oxygen, nutrients and vitality providing energy to the mind, clarity of thought and ease of concentration.

The increased blood flow to the head also stimulates the pituitary gland, considered to be the "master gland", controlling the function of the endocrine system including the thyroid, adrenal gland, ovaries and testes among others. These glands in turn regulate metabolism, growth, blood pressure, sexuality and other fundamental body functions making this pose incredibly potent.

Headstand (hold for 1–5 minutes)

Press the elbows into the floor to lift the shoulders out of the ears and lengthen the sides of the neck, tuck the tailbone and scoop the belly and ribs back to find a straight line in the torso.

If your regular practice does not include headstand, please skip this pose.

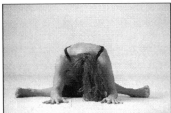

19: Twist (Week Two): Hold for 5-10 breaths each side

20: Pigeon Pose (Week Three): Hold for 10-15 breaths

21: Cow Face Pose (*Gomukhasana*)

Cow face pose is a great for the lateral hips and lower back. The stillness in this pose is nourishing for the kidneys and adrenals and the forward fold stimulates the abdominal organs. Athletes or people who sit at a desk greatly benefit from this pose.

Cow Face Pose (hold for 1–2 minutes each side)

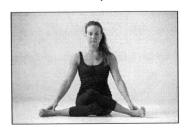
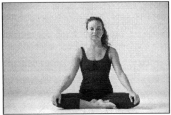
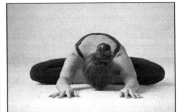

Stack the knees if possible, easier with the feet in closer to the hips, keep the hips reaching back as you walk the hands out, back off or skip if it puts pressure on the knees.

Option: Uncross legs.

22: Savasana (Week One): 3-5 minutes

Take Savasana for 3-5 minutes, then come to a comfortable seated position on a cushion or rolled blanket for meditation.

23: So-Hum Meditation

So-Hum Meditation is a specific technique of meditation that allows the mind to soften through mantra. So-Hum is a yogic mantra meaning: "I am that" (*so* = "I am" and *hum* = "that"). It symbolizes the interconnectedness of everyone and everything.

As you inhale, silently say "so" to yourself and as you exhale, say "hum." At the same time, with the inhale slightly move the right forefinger toward the palm, on the exhale relax the right forefinger away from the palm.

It is best to practice this technique for the first two-thirds of your meditation practice. Sit for the other third.

Day Twenty-Two

As you seek moderation in your diet, keep your eye on eating the right foods and good proteins.

* Read the Proteins section in the Nutrition chapter.

* Set exercise goals for the week.

* Continue your daily yoga practice and the weekly overview tasks.

Here's the breakdown:

Protein Education. Read the Protein section in the Nutrition chapter and start to incorporate this information into your daily eating.

Exercise Goals. Take time today to write down your specific exercise goals for this week.

Exercise and Yoga Goals for This Week		
What	**How many minutes**	**How many times/ week**

Dietary Changes. Continue taking sole, adaptogenic herbs and probiotics, and limit sugar, alcohol, caffeine, wheat and dairy.

Yoga Practice. Follow the yoga sequence described in the Week Four overview.

ॐ **Yoga Index**
For a complete rundown of all poses in this program, please see the Yoga Index.

Day Twenty-Three

Today is a day for taking the time to stop and smell the flowers.

- Buy flowers.
- Reduce your stress.
- Continue your daily yoga practice and the weekly overview tasks.

Here's the breakdown:

Buy Flowers. Buy flowers for your house or office as a reminder to yourself of your commitment as a yogi to make the world a better place by always leaving a person/place a little better than you found them.

Stress Reduction. Below are some techniques for reducing your stress. Try to incorporate one of these on a regular basis when stress creeps into your day.

- **Deep Breathing.** Stress often causes our breathing to be shallow, which causes more stress because it puts less oxygen into the bloodstream and increases muscle tension. This technique can be as simple or as complex as you want to make it. The easiest way is to inhale to a count of six or eight and exhale for the same length, repeat 3-10 times. Try to use this one as soon as you feel the stress creeping in—especially in an acutely stressful situation—to stop the release of harmful stress hormones. This deep breathing technique doesn't have to be an extreme or noticeable event. It simply could be a conscious deepening of the breath without counting as you try to breath down into the belly. Use this technique often. At first it will be difficult to remember, but as you get better at it, you notice the moment the stress symptoms kick in and you will be able to control it quickly. Keep the body relaxed while doing this, especially the shoulders, neck, jaw and forehead.

- **Decompression.** Set aside some time to decompress from your workday. For most people, the best time to do this is on the commute home, whether it be by bus, bike or car. If you work from home, take time to leave the house for a walk when you are finished working to separate the parts of your day so you come back refreshed. During your decompression time, turn off your phone and for at least 10 minutes forget about appointments, tasks or performance, whether related to work, home or relationships. Use this time to relax and observe the state of your body. Are you tense? Is your breathing shallow? Let it go. If music helps you relax, play some relaxing music you enjoy, but try not to let your stress and worries carry your mind away. You'll feel refreshed when you arrive at home and you'll be much more welcome at home if you leave your stress behind.

- **Progressive Muscular Relaxation.** Progressive Muscular Relaxation (PMR) is a technique for relaxing your body when the muscles are tense. The idea behind PMR is that you tense a group of muscles so they are as contracted as possible. You hold them in a state of extreme tension for a few seconds and then relax the muscles even more as you release. You can apply PMR to any or all of the muscle groups in your body depending on whether you want to relax your whole body or just a single area. Experiment with PMR by forming a fist and clenching your hand as tightly as you can for a few seconds. Then consciously relax it so it's as loose as possible. You should feel deep relaxation in the muscles. PMR can be used in conjunction with deep breathing and imagery (see below) for maximum relaxation.

- **Imagery.** Imagery can be a potent method for stress reduction, especially when combined with physical methods such as deep breathing. One common use of imagery in relaxation is to imagine a scene, place or event that you remember as peaceful and restful. Bring all your senses into the image—sounds of running water and birds, the smell of cut grass, the taste of cool crisp water, the feel of the warmth of sun, etc. Use the imagined place as a retreat from stress and pressure. Other uses of imagery in relaxation involve mental pictures of stress flowing out of the body. Use of imagery is as flexible as the effort you put into developing images that meet your specific needs.

- **Relaxation Response.** Here are some steps to induce the relaxation response within the body:

  - Sit quietly in a comfortable position and close your eyes.

  - Deeply relax all your muscles, beginning at your feet and progressing up to your face.

  - Breathing through your nose, become aware of your breathing.

  - As you breathe out, say the word, "one" silently to yourself. For example, breathe in, breathe out and say "one," breathe in, breathe out and say "one," and so on. Breathe easily and naturally.

  - Continue like this for 10-20 minutes. Try not to "watch the clock." When you finish, sit quietly for several minutes with your eyes closed then slowly open your eyes. Take your time standing up and slowly returning to your life.

- Do not worry about whether you are successful in achieving deep relaxation. Keep a passive attitude and just allow relaxation to occur at its own pace. When distracting thoughts occur, try to ignore them by not dwelling upon them and return to repeating "one." With practice, the response should come with little effort. Practice the technique once or twice daily.

- **Positive Reinforcement.** Remember everything that you say to yourself or believe about yourself is imprinted on your cells and affects you mentally, physically and emotionally. Negative thoughts only add to your stress. But thinking positively can greatly change your outlook and reduce your stress levels.

It's best to start practicing positive reinforcement by lying down completely relaxed with your eyes closed. As you get better at it, use it as a mental reminder throughout your day. Use positive reinforcement to visualize yourself confidently executing a previously intimidating task or to reinforce any changes you wish to make in your life, whether physical (weight loss, performance, fertility, pain, energy) or mental/ emotional (confidence, happiness, concentration). Once you are relaxed all you have to do is visualize these changes. For example, see yourself at your optimal weight, notice what it feels like, feel the freedom and new movement your body can explore. Or imagine yourself giving that important presentation with confidence and authority. Observe how calm your body feels, notice the quality of the breath. Many professional athletes use variations of this technique to achieve peak performance.

You can use positive reinforcement with others in mind, too. Visualize people who create stress in your life. Imagine them with their own stress. Then imagine what they would be like without that stress, if they were really happy. You can use this technique with your coworkers , friends and family, if you are struggling with them or if you want to see them happy and healthy. With any of these situations, make sure you use as much detail as possible. Use all your senses and visualize the optimal outcome in detail. Try to be positive and in return show your appreciation for the people around you. Because, as much as we hate to admit it, we are all dependent on each other. Don't be afraid to show your gratitude. The more you put out there the more it will come back around to you.

- **Exercise as Stress Reduction.** Exercise is also a great stress release as long as it's something you enjoy and perceive as a release. Regular exercise is crucial to decreasing your long-term stress levels. The most important thing is to breathe deeply and mindfully to reap all the stress-reducing benefits. If you are doing intense cardio, it may not be possible to keep the breath deep, but mindfully observe the breath so even if it speeds up, it stays smooth and even. Make sure that you're not tensing unnecessary body parts like the shoulders, neck, jaw or forehead. Let me reinforce this once more: exercise is not stress reduction if you are grunting through it, dreading it or tensing the body. Find something you like and enjoy!

- **Other.** Some other options for stress reduction are Tai Chi, Qi Gong, meditation, massage, a hot bath, dance, art, etc. These are just suggestions. If all else fails, be creative and find something that works for you. Anything you enjoy doing that relaxes you and that you approach with the intention of releasing stress will work. The breathing and visualizing techniques seem to create a longer lasting effect due to their ability to reprogram the nervous system and the way that it responds to stress.

Dietary Changes. Continue taking sole, adaptogenic herbs and probiotics, and limit sugar, alcohol, caffeine, wheat and dairy.

Yoga Practice. Follow the yoga sequence described in the Week Four overview.

Day Twenty-Four

Nourishment isn't just about food. It's about feeding the spirit as well.

- Nourish yourself.
- Look at your finances and plan a budget.
- Continue your daily yoga practice the weekly overview tasks.

Here's the breakdown:

Nourish Yourself. Find some way to nourish yourself today that doesn't involve any material objects. Maybe some silence, a bath, a walk with no destination, eating your meal mindful of every bite, drinking your water like each sip is your last, whatever you choose.

Finances and Budget. Today sit down and create a money plan and a budget. Money is one of the most common stressors in modern-day society, so getting straight with your money is of utmost importance to your stress level. Are you happy with where you are at financially? Are you happy with the amount you're saving and putting away for retirement? If you have debts, make a reasonable plan to work your way out of debt. Make sure you are putting away enough money each month and planning ahead for retirement and unexpected expenses. Look at your spending over the past year and notice where you can be more efficient and what areas are deal-breakers. Notice what are good investments (your health, good quality food, etc) and which areas may be a good place to cut back (drinking/eating out, coffee shops, clothes, etc). It is a good yogic practice to look deeply at what you actually need to live your optimal life based on your priorities and goals.

Dietary Changes. Continue taking sole, adaptogenic herbs and probiotics, and limit sugar, alcohol, caffeine, wheat and dairy.

Yoga Practice. Follow the yoga sequence described in the Week Four overview.

Day Twenty-Five

Turn off the television and see possibilities.

- Fast from television.
- Study yoga philosophy.
- Continue your daily yoga practice and the weekly overview tasks.

Here's the breakdown:

Television Fast. Do one last television fast. In the absence of noise and distraction, use this time to deepen your understanding of how yogic philosophy applies to you.

Yoga Philosophy. On Day 18, you read about the Eight Limbs of Yoga and learned about the first four limbs of this ancient philosophy. Today you'll explore the final four limbs, which are all very relevant and applicable to our daily lives. Write in your journal today as to how these last four limbs of yoga apply to your life.

ॐ *The Eight Limbs of Yoga*

1. **Yamas** *(don'ts)*
2. **Niyamas** *(do's)*
3. **Asana**
4. **Pranayama** *(breath/energy control)*

5. **Pratyahara** *(withdrawal of the senses)*

6. **Dharana** *(one-pointed focus)*

7. **Dhyana** *(meditation, sustained focus or absorption)*

8. **Samadhi** *(enlightenment)*

Let's look at these last four limbs more closely.

5. Pratyahara

- *Sense withdrawal*
- *Withdrawal of the mind from external objects and experiences*
- *Shift the awareness from the outer world to the inner world*

6. Dharana

- *One-pointed focus*
- *No sensory disturbances, no restless outward thoughts*

7. Dhyana

- *Meditation*
- *Sustained uninterrupted one-pointed focus*
- *One becomes absorbed into and identified with the object of concentration*

8. Samadhi

- *Enlightenment*
- *Oneness*
- *Complete absorption*
- *The subject-object relationship as well as one's ego is dissolved*
- *There is a perception of oneness with the entire universe*

Dietary Changes. Continue taking sole, adaptogenic herbs and probiotics, and limit sugar, alcohol, caffeine, wheat and dairy.

Yoga Practice. Follow the yoga sequence described in the Week Four overview.

Day Twenty-Six

Work environments can be toxic, too. Today look at how to better position your body while at work.

- Improve your ergonomics.

- Try myofascial release for your shoulders.

- Continue your daily yoga practice and the weekly overview tasks.

Here's the breakdown:

Improve Ergonomics. Because I see so many patients with repetitive motion injuries from computers, this book wouldn't be complete without recommendations about ergonomics. Take time today to check out your computer setup. If you have persistent pain as a result of computer use, get a more thorough evaluation and/or seek care from an acupuncturist, massage therapist or chiropractor. For soft tissue injuries, I also highly recommend a treatment called Active Release Technique (ART). For more information or to find a provider near you go to *www.Active Release.com*

- **General Ergonomics.** Here are some basic ergonomic guidelines for setting up a computer workstation to minimize repetitive strain injuries.

    1. Use a good chair with lumbar support or use a small rolled up towel behind the lower back or back support cushion.

    2. Top of monitor screen should be 2-3 inches above eye level.

    3. No glare on screen.

    4. Sit at arms length from monitor—further if distance is comfortable and screen is readable.

    5. Rest feet on floor or on a stable foot rest.

    6. Use a document holder, preferably in-line with the computer screen.

    7. Wrists flat or slightly flexed to use keyboard/mouse.

    8. Keeps arms and elbows close to body, with shoulders relaxed down away from ears.

    9. Center monitor and keyboard in front of you.

10. Use a negative tilt keyboard tray, with mouse and keyboard down so forearms are parallel to floor with shoulders relaxed.

11. Use a stable work station.

12. Raise or lower your chair height so that there is a 90 to 110-degree angle at your hips, knees and elbows.

13. Adjust chair armrests, in/out or up/down, or remove armrests if they are not used, do not hunch over or lean on them.

14. Take frequent short breaks to stretch.

◆ **Ergonomic Exercises.** After every 30-60 minutes of continuous computer use, pause to perform a few office exercises. These are very simple but very helpful exercises.

✍ **Note: Pain? Do Not Gain**
Do not do any of these exercises if they are painful.

• **Eyes**

• To relieve dry eyes, close your eyes tightly for a second and then open them widely. Repeat several times.

• Hold your index finger up about 6-8 inches in front of you and focus your eyes on your finger, then focus your eyes on an object that is about 10-15 feet away. Repeat several times getting faster so that your eyes are only on the object long enough to bring it into focus. Shift back and forth between objects about a dozen times then close your eyes and rest and repeat 2-3 times.

• **Hands/Forearms**

• Spread your fingers wide and hold, form fists and hold. Repeat several times.

• Place your hands together with fingers pointing upwards and at chin level. Slowly lower your hands, part them and reverse the process. Repeat several times.

• **Neck**

• Keeping your chin tucked in, slowly turn your head to one side and hold.

• Alternate sides and repeat several times.

• **Shoulders**

• Slowly shrug shoulders in a forward circular motion. Alternate to reverse circular motion.

- **Whole Body**
    - While standing, with room around you, inhale reach arms up overhead with a deep breath, exhale folding forward to a comfortable forward fold. Repeat 5-10 times.
    - If all else fails just get up and walk, jumping jacks, handstands, headstands, deep breathing, sun salutations… Just move for 1-3 minutes every 30-60 minutes.

- **Work Environment.** Make changes to your work environment as you notice problems.
    - Cramped leg space? Clear out items beneath the work surface or rearrange your work area.
    - Reaching too far for tools, etc.? Reorganize your work area to allow the most frequently used items to be within a forearm's reach.
    - Avoid frequent reaches above shoulder height.
    - Reduce the need for awkward head movements by placing your documents as close as possible to the computer monitor. Consider using a document holder to improve the viewing angle.

- **Work Practices.** It's not just the equipment that creates ergonomic problems. How you use your body while working affects your comfort too.

    - **Improper work postures?**
        - Avoid sustained, awkward postures.
        - Pay attention to any body discomfort from prolonged positions.

    - **Extended periods of computer use?**
        - As a routine work practice, take a 1-3 minute break after every 30-60 minutes at the computer.
        - Use a timer to remind yourself to take a break.
        - Perform office exercises to relax and to rest eyes.

Myofascial Release. Continue myofascial techniques to release the shoulder and rhomboid muscles.

Lateral Shoulder Release

This is a great practice for shoulder injuries or range of motion as well as low back issues since it works on the lateral muscles and the positioning of the

Optimal Health for a Vibrant Life

shoulder girdle for posture. Great for frozen shoulder, rotator cuff problems, low back pain, poor posture and rounded shoulders. This is also a great preparation for kapotasana or shoulder or back tension in postures with the arms overhead (wheel, drop backs, etc.)

For this one you will prefer a foam roller or a foam yoga block.

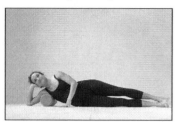

Lie on your side and place your foam roller/block under the outer edge of the armpit and shoulder blade at the upper rib cage. Place the same side hand under your head to support it with your elbow on the floor and place the other hand on the floor in front of you for balance. Slowly tilt you body forward toward your front arm then back toward the wall behind you looking for tender or tight areas and stopping there to breath and relax the area for a minute or two. Then roll a little up or down on the foam roller until you find a good spot and repeat then change sides.

Rhomboid Release

This is a great technique for releasing the rhomboid muscles between the shoulder blades that are often tight from sitting for extended periods—great for people who sit at their computer a lot or those with poor posture.

For this one you will need two tennis balls. Refer to the photo for placement of tennis balls.

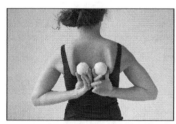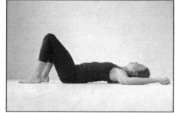
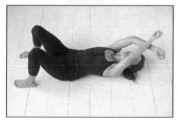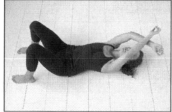

Lie on your back and bend your knees to place your feet on the floor and make sure you have some room to move around here. Lift the hips and place the tennis balls on either side of the spine just below the level of the shoulder blades. Relax completely using the weight of the body to relax the muscles. If you are happy here, slowly begin making circles with the arms as large as you can comfortably. Then walk the hips down a few inches so that the balls are 2–3 inches higher on the back and relax in again. If you're happy here, to slowly cross the arms in front of you and the spread them wide, repeating several times, switching the cross of the arm on top each time. Then walk the hips down a few inches so that the balls are 2–3 inches higher on the back and relax in again.

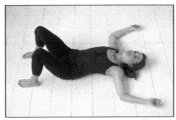
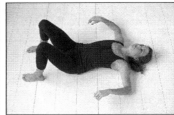

If you're happy here, bring the arms out to the sides with the elbows bent like a cactus. Then you can slowly bring the hands up and over to point overhead and then down to point toward your feet keeping the elbows on the ground.

Rotator Cuff Release

This is a great technique for releasing the rotator cuff muscles, specifically the infraspinatus and teres minor that are often strained in shoulder injuries. This is great for swimmers, yogis, pitchers, tennis players, golfers, discus or javelin throwers and any sport that involves throwing or repetitive movements of the shoulder. Use with the lateral shoulder release and rhomboid release for shoulder injuries.

For this one you will need two tennis balls. Refer to the photo for placement of tennis balls (one shown).

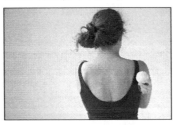
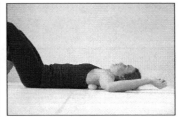
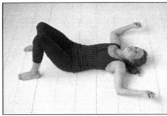
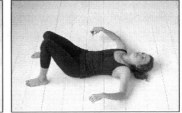

Lie on your back and bend your knees to place your feet on the floor. Make sure you have some room to move around here. Lift the hips and place the tennis balls underneath the shoulder blades so that the shoulder blades rest on top of the balls, using the weight of the body to relax the muscles. Roll around until you find a tender area. Once you are able to relax into it, try bringing the arms out to the sides with the elbows bent like a cactus. If you are comfortable, slowly bring the hands up and over to point overhead and then down to point toward your feet keeping the elbows on the ground. Then move the balls to find another spot and repeat stopping at the tender or tight areas for at least a couple minutes.

Dietary Changes. Continue taking sole, adaptogenic herbs and probiotics, and limit sugar, alcohol, caffeine, wheat and dairy.

Yoga Practice. Follow the yoga sequence described in the Week Four overview.

Day Twenty-Seven

In these last few days, look at and plan to deal with the toxins around you.

- Purchase air and water filters.

- Practice restorative yoga.

- Continue your daily yoga practice and the weekly overview tasks.

Here's the breakdown:

Air and Water Filters. Today research high-quality air and water filters for your house, and maybe your office too, to decrease the amount of toxins your body has to process and eliminate on a daily basis. (I like Ecoquest; I have that brand's Living Water II and the AZ Breeze)

Restorative Yoga. Restorative poses are a great way to relax the musculoskeletal system and reset the nervous system for injuries, stress, anxiety, insomnia, hypertension, indigestion or pain to name a few. The most important thing with these is setting yourself up with enough blocks and props that you can completely relax and be supported here for at least 5 minutes to allow the bones to settle into this new posture to retrain the musculature around the bones to relearn new postural patterns. I recommend picking one or two you like and using them for 5-10 minutes daily to notice the effects.

Restorative Chest Release
This is a great practice for people who sit at a computer a lot, cyclists who lean over their handle bars, or those with poor posture. This is also a great pose for depression, anxiety, asthma or shortness of breath since trigger points in this area often accompany these.

☾ Thought: Gratitude
Use your practice today to express gratitude to yourself and the people around you, for all the wonderful things we have and the amazing potential we each contain.

For this one you will need a foam roller, a thick, tightly rolled up yoga mat, or two yoga blocks.

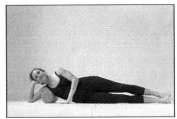 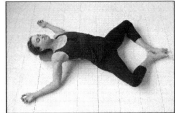

Place the foam roller behind the spine from the back of the head along the length of the spine. The hips will be on the floor but if your foam roller is longer it may extend under the hips if you prefer. Make yourself comfortable here and either extend the legs, bend the knees and put the feet on the floor; or bend the knees and place the soles of the feet together. Arms come out to the sides either straight or bent for more of a stretch, play with the distance from the body by moving the arms up or down to get different segments of the chest muscles. Choose one spot and stay here for 3–5 minutes, completely still so that the weight of the bones draws you in deeper. Use the inhale to breathe into the tight areas and the exhale to relax into it. To come out slowly roll onto one side and press up to seated.

Restorative Mid/Upper Back Release

For this one you will need a foam roller, bolster/roll or yoga block.

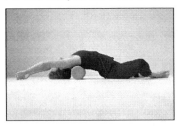 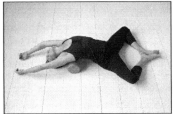

Lie on your back and place the foam roller underneath you horizontally across the mid-back under the lower tips of the shoulder blades. Legs are either extended, bent, up the wall or soles of the feet together. Arms are extended overhead, straight or bent. If you need support for the head place a blanket or pillow there. If you need more support for the lower back, roll a blanket up behind the knees. Stay for 5–10 minutes.

Restorative Hip Opener

For this one you may need a yoga block.

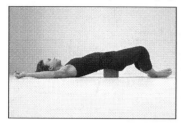 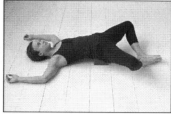

On your back bring the soles of the feet together, using blankets or props to support yourself under your head or knees. To intensify the hip opening place a block under your sacrum and let the legs continue to drop down toward the floor. You can extend the arms out to the sides or place them on your belly and chest. Breathe into your hips for 3–5 minutes. If you're having trouble relaxing use a little proprioceptive feedback to help you relax by lifting the knees an inch higher from the floor to contract the inner thighs and hold for about 5 seconds and then relax in a little deeper and repeat 1–3 times.

Restorative Legs up the Wall

This is a great pose to revive the lower body after a long day of standing and is great for varicose veins. As with all inversions the effects of this pose are numerous and extend to many different organ systems; this supported version allows us to stay longer to deepen the effects of the inversion.

You may need a block or blanket for this one.

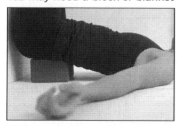 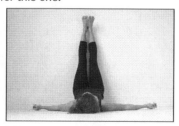

Lie on your side with the knees bent in toward your chest and the hips up against the wall. Then roll onto your back and extend the legs up the wall with the hips as close to the wall as your hamstrings will allow. To intensify the inversion effects place a block or blanket under your hips.

Front Body Restorative

For this one you need two yoga blocks and possibly a yoga strap.

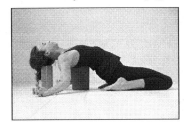 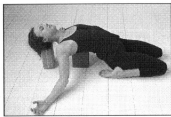

This pose is a little trickier; if it bothers the knees then use one of the previous postures. For this pose, use two blocks and possibly a strap around the knees to keep them together. One block on its middle or highest level goes between the shoulder blades and the other goes under the head. You'll feel opening of the entire front side of the body and mid-back. Hold for 1–5 minutes and then slowly come out and take child's pose.

Dietary Changes. Continue taking sole, adaptogenic herbs and probiotics, and limit sugar, alcohol, caffeine, wheat and dairy.

Yoga Practice. Follow the yoga sequence described in the Week Four overview.

Today for your meditation try this loving kindness meditation. Start by sitting and watching the breath for a few minutes; once you're settled, contemplate each of these for at least 3-5 minutes:

Just as I want happiness and not to suffer, so everyone wants happiness and not to suffer.

Just as I want happiness and not to suffer, so _____(your closest friend) wants happiness and not to suffer.

Just as I want happiness and not to suffer, so _____(someone you don't know) wants happiness and not to suffer.

Just as I want happiness and not to suffer, so _____(an enemy or someone you struggle with) wants happiness and not to suffer.

Day Twenty-Eight

Again, as you look at the world around you, analyze the sum of toxins both external and internal.

• Look at your Total Load.

• Continue your daily yoga practice and the weekly overview tasks.

Here's the breakdown:

Total Load. Today I want you to look at your Total Load. This is a technique I learned from Dr. Frank Lipman, MD, an outstanding doctor I had the pleasure to work with when I was treating patients in New York City. The ideas here are taken from his book *Total Renewal*, which I highly recommend. (His book *Spent* is equally phenomenal.)

- **Decreasing Your Total Load, Potential Burdens.** It's important when we talk about optimal health to realize that you will never be perfect. What's important is that you try to decrease the total load on your system. I have included a list of potential burdens to your system, not as a checklist of all the things you should do, but rather as a way to see what you can change to help lighten the load on your body and in so doing improve your health. Some of these are changeable, others are not and still others may be deal breakers for you. Look over the list and note the things you can change to decrease the Total Load on your system for lasting optimal health.

  - **Environmental Toxins**
    - Outdoor pollution
    - Indoor pollution (carpet, dust, mold/mildew, manufactured wood products)
    - Chemicals in drinking water
    - Chemicals in food (processed food, pesticides, hormones, antibiotics, coloring, preservatives, additives, food packaging, genetically modified foods)
    - Chemicals in personal care products
    - Heavy metals
    - Radiation
    - Noise pollution
  - **Drugs**
    - Prescription
    - Over-the-counter
    - Recreational
    - Stimulants (caffeine)
  - **Allergies**
    - Pollens, grasses, dust mites, animal dander, mold

- **Diet**
  - Trans-fat
  - Sugar
  - Refined products
  - Imbalance of carbohydrates/protein/fats
  - Food Sensitivities
  - Constant dieting, starving yourself
- **Low-Grade Infections**
  - Parasites, yeast, viral
- **Nutritional Deficiencies**
  - Deficiency of digestive enzymes, vitamins/minerals, amino acids, phytonutrients, essential fatty acids, etc.
- **Metabolic Imbalances**
  - Hormonal imbalances
  - Digestive imbalances
  - Chronic Inflammation
- **Physical**
  - Injuries, repetitive stress/strain, tension
- **Work**
  - Too many responsibilities, long hours, not enough time off/down time, boring and unfulfilling tasks, poor physical and /or emotional conditions
- **Psycho-emotional**
  - Low self-esteem, no sense of purpose, lack of joy/love, unable to forgive, judgmental of self and others, helplessness, unable to ask for help, worry, anxiety, guilt-ridden, often fearful, trouble expressing your emotions
- **Social**
  - Lonely, isolated, lack of family support
- **Spiritual**
  - Lack sense of connection to a higher power or purpose, lacking compassion or gratitude, disregarding your intuition

- Lack of sleep

- Lack of exercise

Dietary Changes. Continue taking sole, adaptogenic herbs and probiotics, and limit sugar, alcohol, caffeine, wheat and dairy.

Yoga Practice. Follow the yoga sequence described in the Week Four overview. Maintain your commitment to a regular yoga practice to revitalize yourself daily. Continue the loving kindness meditation today as described in Day 27.

Day Twenty-Nine

As you move forward this week continue to minimize processed foods and sugars as well as alcohol and caffeine. Moderation is often the hardest part in our all-or-nothing society. It's important to limit the foods that put a damper on the metabolic process but at the same time be able to go out with friends and enjoy yourself from time to time. Remember our mind plays a large role in our mental and physical health; slow down and feel nourished by your food rather than eating mindlessly.

Continue your commitment to your yoga practice, whatever it may be. Remember that life ebbs and flows, so that even if you miss a couple days or a week or two, your health is always there to come back to. Allow yourself to take breaks—from work or kids or yoga—so that you can come back refreshed and renewed, whether it's for a few minutes or a couple weeks. Most of all, this program teaches you what it's like to feel good so that you want to take care of yourself going forward.

- Review your goals and priorities of previous weeks and set new ones for the weeks ahead.

- Continue your daily yoga practice the weekly overview tasks.

Here's the breakdown:

Goals and Priorities. Today review your goals and priorities, including your specific exercise goals (next page). Put a reminder on your calendar to review your goals and priorities once a month.

Dietary Changes. Continue to minimize sugar, alcohol, caffeine and processed foods, focusing on whole foods that will sustain and nourish you. Maintain your commitment to a regular yoga practice to revitalize yourself daily. If you choose you can also continue taking adaptogenic herbs or any of the many other practices we have explored this month.

Goals and Priorities

Take a couple of minutes today to sit down and write out your goals. Then write your priorities based on your goals. Before you begin, answer the following questions. Use a separate sheet of paper so you can update your responses in the future.

1.	What are the five things you value the most in life?
2.	In 30 seconds write: what are the three most important goals in your life right now?
3.	What would you do if you won a million dollars?
4.	What if you only had six months to live? What would your priorities be?
5.	What have you always wanted to do but been afraid to attempt?
6.	What gives you your greatest feeling of importance or purpose?
7.	What one great thing would you dare to dream if you knew you couldn't fail?

Goals

Lifetime: When you look back from your deathbed, what will have made you the happiest?

Ten years: What do you want to accomplish in 10 years?		
One year: What do you want to accomplish this year?		
One month: What do you want to accomplish this month?		

Priorities

Fill in the chart below with your priorities, based on your goals from the previous section, then rank them in importance.

What	Very High	High	Medium
Improve my health			

Ongoing Contract: Optimal Health Program

Reasons for Continuing Optimal Health

Fill out the chart to set your intention for your health and detox program.

1.	
Why	
2.	
Why	
3.	
Why	
4.	
Why	
5.	
Why	

This contract is a commitment to myself and to my quality of my life, which means changing my life. If I am having trouble incorporating something or if doing so seems overwhelming, I will modify it in my goals for the week to make it more attainable for me or find a way to ease into the changes more slowly. I realize that at first some of these changes may seem very difficult. This is because we are creatures of habit. If I stick with making these changes, slowly over time they will become my new habits. A strong awareness of my body and mind is key to my success.

I agree to dedicate myself to incorporating these self-guided changes into my life little by little, following the outline I have been given, knowing that lasting results are in my hands. I realize that my results are dependent upon my efforts and my dedication to a long-term goal. I seek progress rather than perfection. I will review the above goals as often as needed to remind myself of my purpose. I realize that living healthy means changing my habits, lifestyle and my mind set and that it is an ongoing process rather than an endpoint.

Signature	Date
Printed Name	

Yoga Practice. Follow the yoga sequence described in the Week Four overview. Maintain your commitment to a regular yoga practice to revitalize yourself daily. Continue the loving kindness meditation today as described in Day 27.

Day Thirty

It's the last day of the program, but the beginning of your commitment to a healthier, more vibrant life. Look over what worked best for you and come up with a plan, focusing on whole foods and regular meals with protein and veggies.

- Review and sign the Ongoing Contract: Optimal Health Program.

- Continue your daily yoga practice and the weekly overview tasks.

Here's the breakdown:

Ongoing Contract. In Week One, you made a commitment to yourself by signing a Start-Up Contract for this Optimal Health Program. Today, fill out and sign the contract for your health going forward (see opposite page).

Yoga Practice. Follow the yoga sequence described in Week Four overview. Maintain your commitment to a regular yoga practice to revitalize yourself daily. Continue the loving kindness meditation today as described in Day 27.

Congratulations! You're on your way to a healthier, more vibrant future!

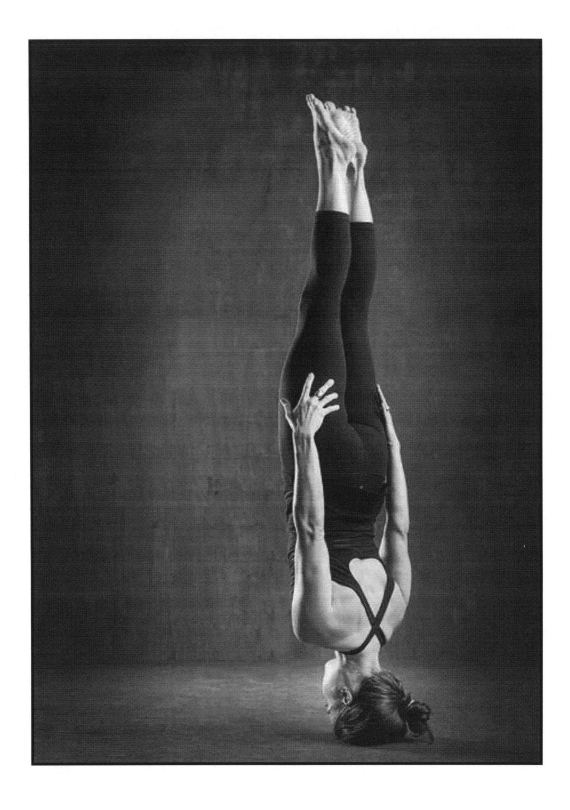

Conclusion

O ver the past 30 days you tried many different detox techniques and you discovered many that are quite therapeutic when used just by themselves. As you move forward you can't help but be more conscious of the food you eat. But it's a good practice to pull out something simple from this book every so often as a refresher. I recommend doing a more thorough detox once or twice a year using several of the techniques we've covered.

Try honing in on a few areas that gave you the most results so that you can incorporate them into your life. For some people simply eliminating wheat and sugar can create a powerful transformation physically and mentally; others love the tinctures, meditation or myofascial release. The most important part of this detox program is learning what works for your body and the effects of these detox techniques so you can use them as needed in the future.

The best changes are the ones that are cultivated over time; 30 days is a great start. Your taste buds changed as you adjusted your palate to what your body needs. Please remember that many of us have spent years accumulating toxins in our bodies. Don't expect a brand new body over night. We are all healthy inside. It's just a matter of how well we've covered it up over the years. How well we covered up our health will often determine how quickly we see changes.

Continue the positive attribute affirmations you began on Day 4 in Week One. These will help you rewire your brain to see yourself in a new perspective to change how you see yourself and to change your life. It takes 21 days to create a new habit so pick one attribute and stick with it for at least 21 days. Then pick another.

It's important to remember that less is more. When we're busy or stressed sometimes, slowing down and doing less can be more potent than a full yoga practice or a full detox. There are many ways to nourish ourselves, including the often-overlooked practice of non-doing. That doesn't mean sitting in front of the television, however. We can nourish ourselves by cooking a simple meal, practicing yoga, taking a warm bath, going for a relaxing walk or by simply sitting and meditating.

The most important part is to move forward with a clear intention, priorities and goals. Just as you go to your yoga mat with an active intention to nourish yourself, the outcome is dramatically different than a practice without intention. Each day set your intention. I find the best time to do so is before I get out of bed, but also before I begin my yoga or at the beginning of a meal.

Life is beautiful! Don't forget to stop and notice.

Now is when everything happens!

For more information and resources go to *www.TiffanyYoga.com.*

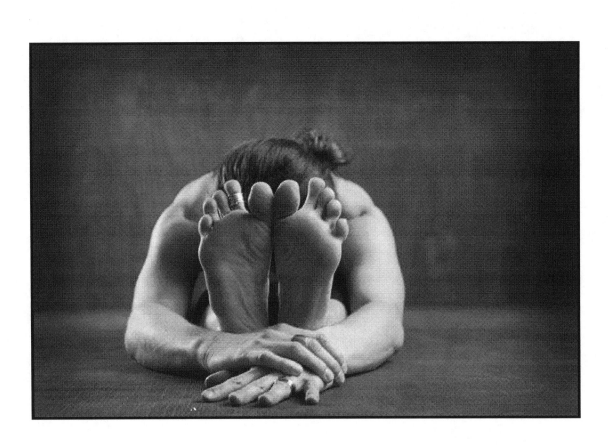

Resources

"An emotion is the body's reaction to your mind."
— Eckhart Tolle, *The Power of Now*

ॐ Yoga Index

All the yoga poses in this book at a glance, shown in the final order in which they are practiced in Week Four. For complete instructions, refer to the week in which they were introduced.

1: Pranayama: Weeks One–Four

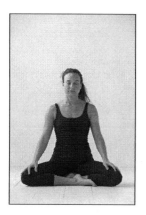

2: Cat/Cow (*Marjarasana*): Week One

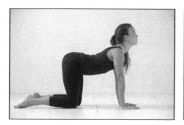 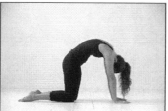 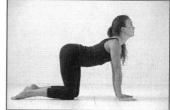

3: Tabletop with Stability Work: Week One

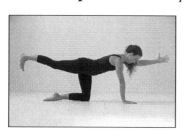

4: Sun Salutation (*Surya Namaskara*), Version A: Week One

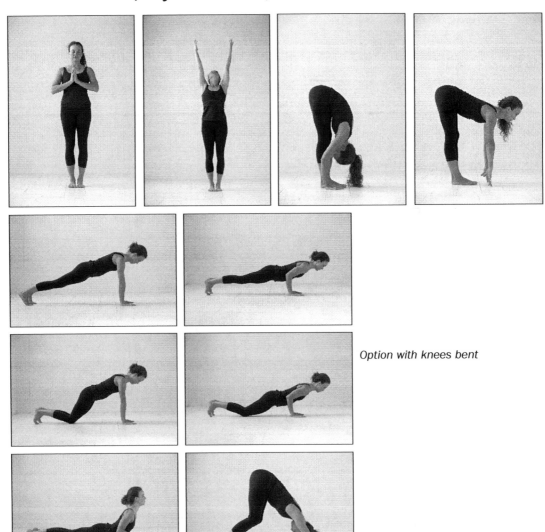

Option with knees bent

Optimal Health for a Vibrant Life

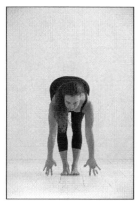 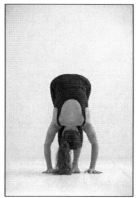 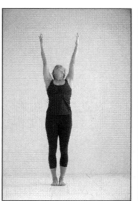 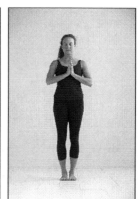

5: Sun Salutation (*Surya Namaskara*), Version B: Week One

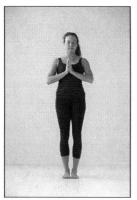 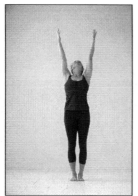 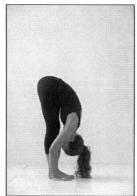 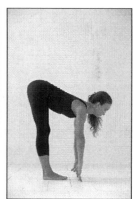

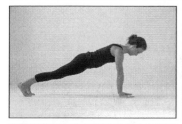 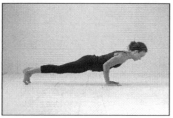

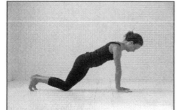 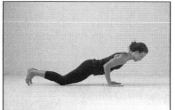

Option with knees bent

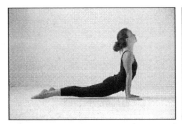
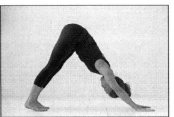

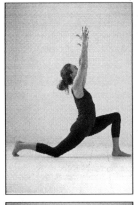
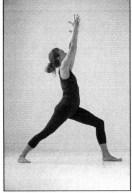
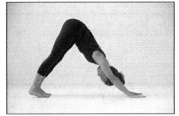

Or Vinyasa

Option with straight leg

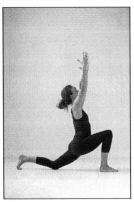
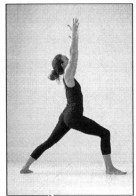
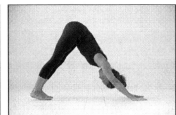

Or Vinyasa

Option with straight leg

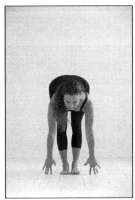
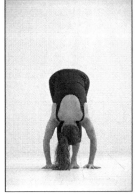
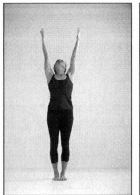
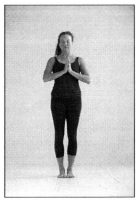

Optimal Health for a Vibrant Life

6: Chair Pose and Twist (*Utkatasana and Parivritta Utkatasana*): Week Four

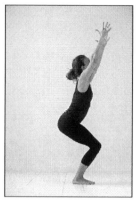 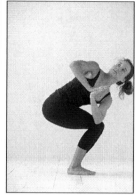

7. Triangle Pose (*Trikonasana*): Week Two

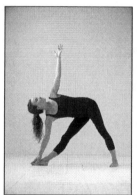 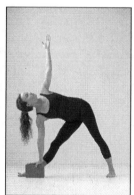 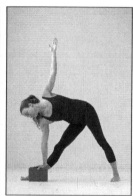

Options with block

8: Revolved Triangle (*Parivrtta Trikonasana*): Week Two

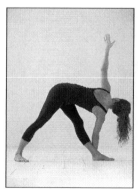 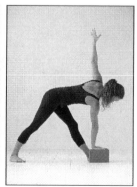

Option with block

9: Extended Side Angle Pose (*Utthita Parsvakonasana*): Week Three

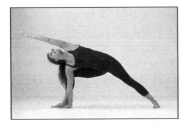
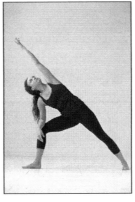

Option with arm on knee

10: Half Moon (*Ardha Chandrasana*): Week Four

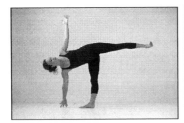
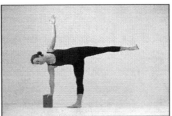

11. Locust Pose (*Salabhasana*): Week Three

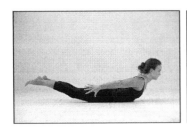
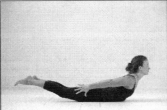

12: Camel Pose (*Utrasana*): Week Four

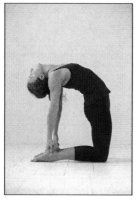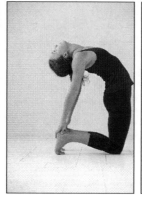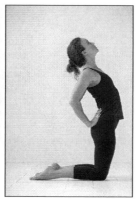

Options with toes turned under or with hands on sacrum

13: Boat Pose (*Navasana*): Week Two

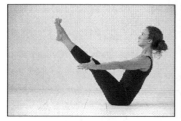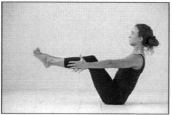

Option with knees bent

14: Bridge Stability: Week Four

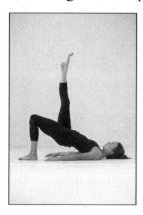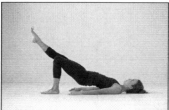

15: Bridge Pose (*Setu Bandhasana*): Week Two

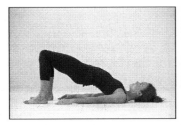 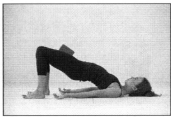

16: Shoulder Stand (*Sarvangasana*): Week Three

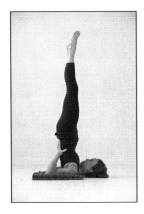

17: Fish Pose (*Matsyasana*)Week Three:

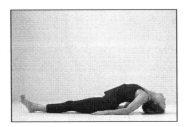

18: Headstand (*Shirshasana*): Week Four

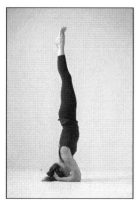

Optional pose: do only if experienced

19: Twist (*Supta Matsyendrasana*): Week Two

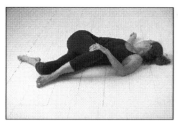 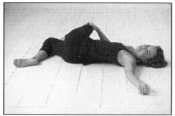

20: Pigeon Pose (*Eka Pada Rajakpotasana*): Week Three

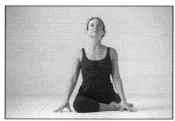 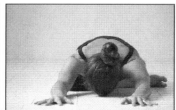 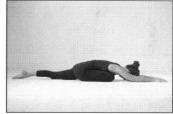

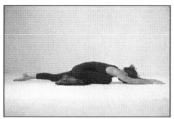

Option with folded blanket

21: Cow Face Pose (*Gomukhasana*): Week Four

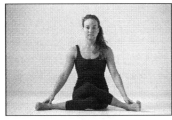
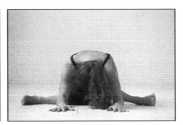
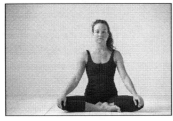
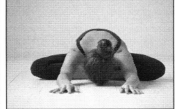

Option with legs uncrossed

22: Savasana: Week One

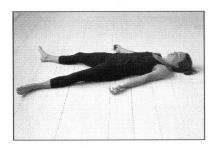

23: Meditation: Weeks One–Four

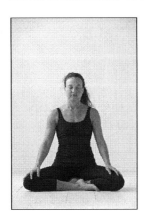

🍽 Recipes

Sauces, Dressings, Dips and Marinades

Raw Vegan Sour Cream Sauce/Dip/Dressing

2 cups soaked almonds (soak overnight in water, then drain)
2 Tbls lemon juice
1 clove garlic
1 tsp sea salt
1 tsp cumin
1 tsp black pepper
1-3 cups water (depends on if you want it thick like sour cream or thin for a dressing or dip, maybe start thick and add more to vary it from the thicker base so you can use it for different things throughout the week)

Blend until smooth and creamy, optional- stir in finely chopped green onions at the end. This one is great as a dip for veggies, etc.

Tamari Ginger Marinade

½ cup sake
½ cup Mirin
½ cup Tamari or natural soy sauce
1 Tbls fresh grated ginger
2 clove garlic smashed

Mix sake, Mirin, Tamari, ginger and garlic together and soak fish (salmon, cod…) at least 1-3 hours, even better overnight.

Miso Marinade, Sauce or Dressing

¼ cup Mirin
1 Tbls of Miso
1 Tbls of honey
¼ cup Sake (optional, only if using to cook, not for dressings)
Rice vinegar and Olive or sesame oil (optional, for dressings)

This is a base for many things, start playing, taste as you go to see how much of each you like!

Citrus Sauce, Dressing or Marinade

Juice of ½-1 lemon or lime
1 tsp of honey
Vinegar (apple cider, balsamic, rice, white/red wine vinegar…)
Mix these, then add

Olive oil (add slowly and mix as you add it)
Sea Salt to taste
This is a good base, you can add and herbs or spices or mustard or horse-
radish or leave out the lemon, etc. Play, have fun!

Orange Shallot Dressing/Sauce

In blender mix

½ Tbls minced shallot
½ cup fresh squeezed orange juice
While blending slowly add

1 cup Olive Oil
Blend until it thickens and becomes creamy colored, then add

1 Tbls fresh lemon juice
1 Tbls honey
½ tsp black pepper
½ tsp sea salt or to taste

Miso Orange Dressing/Sauce

Blend

½ cup fresh squeezed orange juice
½ cup olive oil or flax oil
⅛ cup lemon juice
2 Tbls miso

Curry Carrot Dressing/sauce

Blend until creamy

2 carrots, chopped
2 Tbls sesame oil
1 Tbls ginger, peeled and minced
1½ tsp curry
¼ tsp nutmeg

Lemon Ginger Dressing

Blend until smooth

½ cup olive oil

⅓ cup fresh lemon juice

3 Tbls Tamari or Braggs

¹/₆ cup water

1 Tbls fresh ginger peeled and sliced

1½ Tbls sunflower seeds

1 tsp dry mustard

1 clove garlic, peeled

Cucumber-Yogurt Sauce

3 cups plain whole milk greek style yogurt

1 cucumber (about 16 ounces), peeled, halved lengthwise, seeded

1 large garlic clove, minced

Transfer yogurt to medium bowl. Coarsely grate cucumber and place in a strainer over a bowl; let stand at room temperature until most of liquid drains out, about 1-3 hours. Discard liquid. Squeeze excess moisture from cucumber. Mix cucumber and garlic into yogurt. Cover and refrigerate (best made 1 day ahead to sit in fridge and soak up the flavor)

Macadamia Cream Sauce/Dip/Dressing

Blend until creamy, about 30 seconds

½ cup macadamia nuts

3 Tbls lemon juice

¼ cup coconut water (*from white young coconuts, found in most natural foods stores in whole form or the coconut water can usually be bought in a small one serving size beverage in the refrigerated beverage area*)

This sauce makes an excellent dip for veggies or crackers! A great snack to have in the fridge that will satiate you without all the carbs to make you sleepy.

Walnut Spread

Blend

2 cups walnuts, soaked overnight

1 cup leek, finely chopped

2 Tbls olive oil or to your consistency

1 Tbls Italian or other seasoning

1 tsp sea salt

Add water or olive oil as needed for consistency.

Pumpkin Seed Dip

Blend

    2 cups pumpkin seeds, soaked overnight
    ½ cup sun-dried tomatoes, soaked 20-30 minutes
    2 Tbls olive oil or to the consistency you like
    1 Tbls fresh parley, minced
    1 Tbls lemon juice
    1 tsp fresh oregano, minced
    1 tsp fresh thyme, minced
    1 tsp sea salt

Entrees and Salads

Sautéed Garbanzo Bean Recipe (Vegan)

    3 tablespoons coconut oil
    2 15-ounce cans garbanzo beans, drained
    ½ cup onions, diced
    ½-¾ cup of broth
    1 cup kale, chopped
    1 teaspoon cumin
    1 teaspoon chili powder
    ½ teaspoon sea salt
    1 cup diced tomatoes

In a large skillet, heat oil and sauté onions for 2 minutes, stirring as you go. Add garbanzo beans and sauté 7 minutes more, stirring frequently. Add broth, kale, cumin, chili powder and salt, and cook uncovered on low to medium heat for 5 minutes Add tomatoes, mix well and serve.

Thai Cucumber Salad

Combine salt and cucumber then set in a strainer for about an hour

    2 cucumbers thinly sliced
    Just shy of a tsp of sea salt
Add and mix together

    ⅓ cup sesame oil
    1½ Tbls lime juice
    1½ Tbls fresh basil, finely chopped
    ⅓ Tbls fresh ginger, minced
    ⅓ cup leeks finely chopped(optional)

Rainbow Salad

Rinse and dry

> Mixed greens
> Peel and grate
> Daikon
> Burdock
> Beet
> Carrot
> (Or any combination of these)

Add

> Yellow bell peppers, chopped or sliced
> Tomato, chopped or sliced
> Avocado, chopped
> Any nuts or seeds

Combine all above then add to taste

> Lemon juice (approximately ½)
> Apple cider vinegar (approximately 1-2 tsp)
> Olive oil (generous with)
> Sea salt (large pinch or two)

So good, so healthy, a great cleansing salad with lots of vitamins, minerals and antioxidants!

Satiating Snack

> 1 avocado, chopped
> 1 tomato, chopped
> 1 lime-juice
> Sea Salt

Or

> 1 avocado, chopped
> 1 tomato, chopped
> 1 Tbls or so of fresh chopped basil
> Balsamic vinegar, olive oil and sea salt to taste

Combine, stir and enjoy! This is a great snack because it's quick and easy and has some healthy fats to satiate you and give you a more steady fuel than the quick carbs we might normally reach for.

Blended Broccoli Soup

In large soup pan sauté, 1-2 minutes until translucent

    1 Tbls coconut oil
    2 medium green onions, coarsely chopped
    2 cloves garlic, minced
    Stir in over medium heat until bright green
    Large head fresh broccoli, chopped

Add and cover for 3-4 minutes, until bright green

    2 cups your choice of kale or collard greens
    1 Tbls basil, dried

Transfer to food processor or blender with a little broth, then add remainder of broth

    4 cups vegetable or chicken broth
    2 cups coconut milk
    1 tsp sea salt
    Couple dashes of hot sauce

Enjoy!

Dandelion

Dandelion is a very nutritious leafy green, great for cleansing the liver and high in minerals. It can be a little bitter, but with the right preparation it can make a delicious detox salad.

Dandelion Detox Salad

    Mix salad together and set aside
    1 cup dandelion greens, finely chopped (if the stems are thick you
       can remove them to lessen the bitterness)
    1 cup romaine lettuce, chopped
    ½ cup parsley
    ½ cup pine nuts
    Optional any other veggies you want-bell pepper is good, add the
    Miso Orange Dressing

Dandelion Cream Salad

Finely chop a head of dandelion (remove the main stem)

Massage (yes massage, the salt breaks down the fiber) dandelion leaves with 1 tsp sea salt and let sit at least 5 minutes

Then add the Macadamia Cream Sauce/Dip/Dressing

Pour over salad and add

¼ cup red bell pepper or other veggies

Baked Quinoa-Falafel Sandwiches with Cucumber Yogurt Sauce

For the Cucumber Yogurt Sauce, see Sauce recipes.

Falafel Patties

1½-2 cups cooked quinoa slightly cooled
3 cups cooked organic chickpeas (if using canned, discard liquid and rinse thoroughly with cool water)
½ cup green onions, roughly chopped
½ cup chopped fresh cilantro or Italian flat leaf parsley
⅓-½ cup water
2 Tbls all purpose flour
1 Tbls ground cumin
1 tsp baking powder
¾ tsp salt
¼-½ tsp ground red pepper
3 garlic cloves
Coconut oil to grease the baking sheet

Combine chickpeas and the next 9 ingredients (through garlic) in a food processor; pulse 10 times or until well blended and smooth (mixture will be wet). Spoon chickpea mixture into a large bowl; stir in cooked quinoa starting with one cup and gradually folding in more to reach desired texture. You should be able to form patties; they will be fragile but should hold their form.

Divide mixture into equal portions (about ¼ cup each); shape each portion into a ¼-inch-thick patty. Place patties on a baking sheet coated with coconut oil. Bake at 425° for 10 minutes on each side or until browned. Spread sauce onto an Eze-kiel Tortilla wrap, bread, or pita. Top with falafel patties, tomato slices, cucumber, lettuce or any other veggies you desire!

Black Bean Quinoa Salad

    3 cups cooked quinoa, cooled slightly.

    1 cup canned organic black beans; liquids discarded and thoroughly rinsed

    1 cup diced organic tomatoes

    ¼ cup chopped fresh cilantro or green onion (optional)

    ½ cup fresh mild pico de gallo or other fresh chunky salsa

    Finely chopped fresh jalapeno (to taste, depending on how hot you like it! Avoid the seeds for less heat)

    1 tsp salt

    ½ tsp black pepper (to taste)

    Shredded green leaf and red leaf lettuces, combined.

    Avocado Slices

    Fresh limes

Combine quinoa and the next ingredients through black pepper, Folding together gently so as not to break and smash the beans and tomatoes too much. Place 3/4 cup Quinoa/black Bean mixture atop 2 cups of the lettuce mixture, layer on 4 to 5 slices of avocado and squeeze on some fresh lime juice. Try adding more salsa for extra flavor and some jarred jalapeno slices if you like it spicy.

Grilled Peanut Butter and Banana Sandwich

    One slice flourless Ezekiel Sprouted grain bread

    Almond Butter or coconut butter

    1 thinly sliced or mashed banana

    A little butter or coconut oil to grease your frying pan

Spread almond butter/coconut butter generously on a slice of bread. Pile on the banana slices or spoon on your banana mash. Cook "grilled cheese style" over medium-low heat in a frying pan or skillet coated with a little butter or coconut oil. Cook until lightly browned and warmed through. Maybe save some for a snack later.

Sprouted Almonds

Place almonds in small bowl and add water to cover, let soak over night up to 24 hours, then rinse and drain water and eat, store in fridge in airtight jar in fridge, best eaten in a couple days. Almonds can be difficult to digest because of an enzyme-inhibiting substance in their brown coating. Soaking or sprouting removes this inhibitor so that the enzymes secreted during digestion can do their job.

Carrot Avocado Curry Soup

Blend until smooth and creamy, then heat to your liking

3 cups carrot, chopped
2 cups water
2 avocados chopped
1 clove garlic
3 tsp finely grated ginger or ginger juice
1 tsp lemon juice
1 tsp curry powder
½ tsp cumin
½ tsp sea salt or to taste
¼ tsp cayenne
¼ tsp black pepper

Sweet Carrot Soup

Blend until creamy and heat to your liking

2 carrots chopped
2 stalks celery chopped
2 cups soaked almonds (1 day in water)
2-3 cloves garlic
2 cups water
1½ cup fresh squeezed orange juice
1 tsp nutmeg

Zen Salad

Rinse, then massage cabbage with salt and let sit 10 minutes

2 cups green cabbage
1 tsp sea salt

Add

¼ cup sesame seeds
2 Tbls sesame oil
1 tsp lemon juice

Quinoa Tabouli

In bowl place

4 cups parsley finely chopped
¼ -½ cup quinoa
2 cucumbers, finely chopped

Blend

>4 medium lemons juiced
>½ cup olive oil
>2 tsp dried or fresh mint
>1½ tsp sea salt
>1 tsp black pepper

Pour half the dressing over the parsley/quinoa/cucumber mix and let soak for 30 minutes, then add the rest to your liking and toss, use as a side dish or over lettuce or add more quinoa and make it a seasoned quinoa instead of tabouli.

Breakfast Quinoa with Apples

Place

>1 cup cooked quinoa
>2 cups water
>One chopped apple

In a saucepan and bring to a boil. Reduce to low, cover pan and simmer until quinoa is tender (approximately. 15 minutes) Remove from heat stir in

>Orange zest (½ tsp)
>½ tsp cinnamon

Or you can substitute quinoa flakes and follow directions on the box, adding in the apple while it is cooking, then add in the other ingredients at the end. You can also play with adding almond butter or some raw honey. Eat with Almond Milk, top with some sliced almonds or walnuts.

Lemon Quinoa

>1 cup quinoa
>2 cups water
>1½ tablespoons olive oil
>1 teaspoon grated lemon zest
>2 teaspoons fresh lemon juice

Wash quinoa in 3 changes of cold water in a bowl, draining each time.

Cook quinoa in a medium pot of boiling salted water, cover and simmer, until water is gone and quinoa is dry and fluffy, about 15 minutes. Fluff with a wooden spoon. Transfer quinoa to a bowl and stir in oil, zest, lemon juice and ¼ teaspoon sea salt.

Curried Peanut Soup

In soup pan over medium heat cook until translucent

1 Tbls butter
2 medium garlic cloves, minced
1 cup onions chopped
1 inch slice ginger root, chopped

Add and cook about 3-5 minutes

1 tsp sea salt
1½ Tbls curry powder
½ tsp cumin
½ tsp allspice
2 cups cauliflower, chopped
2 cups bok choy, leaf and stem chopped

Stir in

¾ cup of broth gradually into ½ cup peanut or almond butter until smooth

Add

1 ¼ cup broth to vegetables
Stir in diluted peanut/almond butter and heat for 3-5 minutes
   or until heated through

Stir in

1 Tbls currants, finely minced
¼ tsp or to taste, cayenne or red pepper
1½ cups almond milk

Heat and serve.

Mashed "Potatoes"

Steam until tender in steamer or small amount of water in pan

1 head cauliflower

Blend cauliflower with

2 Tbls organic or raw butter
¼ cup organic or raw half and half
¼ tsp sea salt
Pepper to taste

Brussels Sprout Combo

Over medium/high heat, cook for a few seconds

> 2 Tbls coconut oil
> 2 medium garlic cloves, smashed

Then add for 2-3 minutes or until leeks start to wilt

> 2 medium leeks, sliced

Add for 2-3 minutes

> 4 cups brussels sprouts, stemmed and quartered
> 1 tsp fresh or dried rosemary

Reduce heat to medium/low, stir in

> 1 bunch kale, stems removed and chopped
> ¼ cup water

Cover for 3 minutes, until tender

Remove cover, stir in to coat

> 3 Tbls Dijon mustard

Enjoy!

Spicy Nut Broccoli

Lightly steam broccoli in steamer or small amount of water in pan

> 2 large heads of broccoli, chopped
> Blend (until fairly creamy, do not over blend)
> ¼ cup almond butter
> ¼ cup toasted sesame oil
> ⅛ cup raisins, soaked until soft (20-30 minutes)
> 7 kefir lime leaves, chopped or crumbled
> 1 Tbls ginger, peeled and chopped
> Cayenne pepper to taste

Add the desired amount to broccoli then add
> Sesame seeds
> Purple cabbage (finely chopped) as garnish

Kale Salad

Kale is one of the most nutrient-dense items you can buy.

Remove main stem and chop
    1 bunch lacinato kale
Massage with 1 tsp sea salt until kale wilts, then add
    2 tsp lemon juice and massage again
Add

    1 large tomato, cut or chopped
    ¼ cup olives
Blend until creamy and use as dressing

    1 avocado
    1 stalk celery
    2 Tbls olive oil

Seaweed

Adds a lot of nutrition, just add a pinch to salads or entrees. I just like to keep some soaking in the fridge. My favorites are arame or hijiki, buy it in the bulk bins at most natural food stores. Just add to small bowl and cover with water for a minimum of 10 minutes, you can leave it soaking for a couple days in the fridge, just take a pinch at a time and shake water off and add to meals.

Teas and Beverages

Basic Breakfast Smoothie

    1 scoop of pure whey protein powder or rice protein powder
    Couple scoops of organic plain, whole milk yogurt (optional)
    Banana and peanut butter or almond butter or fresh or frozen fruit
    Milk to taste (almond, oat or rice milk preferably)

Blend and enjoy or take on the go!

Tension Tea

    ½ part Lavender
    1 part Scullcap
    1 part Lemon Verbena
    ½ part Passion flower
Mix together and use 1 tsp per 1 cup of water, let steep for 5 minutes, strain and drink. Relaxes the muscles, soothes the nerves and lifts your mood.

Basic Kombucha Tea Recipe

1. Bring to light boil 3+ quarts filtered water.

2. Add tea: 5-7 tea bags or 2-3 tsp loose tea.

3. Steep 15 minutes, then remove or strain.

4. Add Sugar ½ cup sugar or honey

5. Allow to cool to room temperature, keep covered.

6. Add kombucha strain (which is also at room temperature)

7. Add 2 cups Previously Fermented Kombucha Brew as a Starter, use the liquid that came with the mushroom starter or use ¼ cup white distilled vinegar (to reduce the pH and protect the ferment from pathogens).

8. Cover with a clean cloth, paper towel or coffee filter and a rubber band, set aside in a quiet undisturbed spot. Every time the liquid is disturbed the mushroom will have to start forming over again and not form properly.

9. Ferment. 6-8 days normal brew cycle at 80 °F constant temperature, (8-14 days in the 70s). 60° F or below is not recommended. First time may take longer. Temperature Range: 68°-83° F. Should be sparkling semi-sweet cidery taste. Bottle and leave out at room temperature for another 7-14 days to give it more of a kick or bottle and put directly in the fridge.

10. Save 1-2 cups to begin another batch. Each batch should produce another mushroom. Save one mushroom and tea safely away in the event of some disaster. Use either mushroom to start another batch. You may also combine mushrooms or give away to friends.

There are many various to this recipe, but this is the most basic, you can use flavored teas or add fresh ginger slices or fresh juice when you bottle it then leave it out for 7-14 days with the lid on before putting in the fridge. Once you've tried this basic variation play with others, there are many good recipes online.

Detox Lemonade:

32 oz. (4 cups) filtered water in a glass jar

Juice of 1-2 lemons to taste

Liquid stevia to taste (1-6 drops depending on your preference)

Add the lemon juice and stevia and drink it throughout the day for a sweet reminder to drink your water and add a little extra detox to your day.

Detox Lemonade Tea

    1 Tbls Burdock Root
    1 Tbls Dandelion Root
    32 oz. (4 cups) filtered water
    Juice of 1-2 lemons to taste (optional)
    32 oz. or more glass jar

Each day you will brew your tea for the day (or you can make it the evening before and store in fridge until the next morning, add the lemon juice just before you're ready to drink it though) and drink it throughout the day. To prepare place 32 oz. (4 cups) of cool filtered water in a pot and add the herbs to the water. Bring to a boil and simmer for 10 minutes. Turn off heat and let sit for 5 minutes, then strain the herbs out and place liquid in glass jar. Let cool, add back enough water to make 32 oz., then add lemon juice, stir and drink at room temperature. Use daily for 1-4 weeks for optimal detox effects, then discontinue until your next detox.

Stevia Lemonade

    Large water bottle (32 oz.) full of water
    1-2 lemons/limes juiced
    Stevia drops to taste (3-5 drops usually)

This is a great detox lemonade as well as a great way to get all your water in for those of you that get bored with plain water.

Desserts

Carob Fudge

Blend

    1 cup carob powder
    ½ cup almonds, soaked overnight
    ½ cup coconut oil
    ½ tsp vanilla
    2 dried apricots, soaked 30 minutes, minced

Spread ½ inch thick in 4x7 pan, refrigerate until fudge-like consistency, cut into squares

Mint Whip

Blend until creamy

> 1 apple
> ¾ avocado
> ¼ cup coconut water or to desired consistency
> 1 drop peppermint oil (only 1 drop)
> ¼ cup Goji berries (optional-for sweetness and color)

Chill and serve cool if you like

Monster Cookie Balls

Mix

> 2 cups rolled oats
> 2 eggs
> 1 cup water
> ½ stick of butter, softened

Stir in

> 1 cup nut butter of your choice
> 1 large apple, finely chopped
> ¾ cup raisins or currants
> ½ cup carob chips (optional)
> 2 tsp stevia powder

Form into balls and place a pecan on top, place on lightly greased cookie sheet, bake 10-12 minutes at 350°.

Stevia Tapioca

Combine in medium saucepan and let sit 5 minutes to soften

> 3 Tbls minute tapioca
> 2¼ cups almond milk

Thoroughly whip in

> 1 egg, lightly beaten
> Dash of sea salt

Bring to a low boil, stirring constantly, remove from heat and cool 15 minutes.
Mix together, then stir into previous ingredients:

> ½ cup yogurt
> ½ tsp stevia powder
> 1¼ tsp vanilla extract
> Sprinkle ¼ cup walnuts on top

Sweet Almond Cookies

Preheat oven to 325°

Blend to a coarse meal

    1⅓ cup almonds (add slowly while blender is running)

In a bowl mix together almonds from above with

    1⅓ cup unsweetened shredded coconut
    ½ tsp baking soda
    ½ tsp salt
    ¾ tsp nutmeg

In a small bowl mix together

    3 Tbls dried currants
    3 Tbls dried cherries, chopped into small pieces
    1 large egg
    ½ cup yogurt
    3 Tbls maple syrup
    ½ tsp vanilla

Add to the dry mixture and mix. Drop by spoonfuls onto greased cookie sheet and flatten. Bake 10-20 minutes until golden, watch carefully.

Coconut Macaroons

Preheat oven to 350°, lightly grease cookie sheet (butter)

Blend until well combined

    2 cups shredded coconut (unsweetened)
    ½ cup quinoa flakes
    2 tsp liquid lecithin (flavorful and nutrient-rich, adds a creamy
       quality, found in health food stores)
    2 Tbls salted butter, softened
    ⅛ tsp white stevia powder (or 2 Tbls of agave nectar or honey-but
       add in when you add the egg whites at the end)
    Blend until stiff peaks form
    4 egg whites
    $^1/_{16}$ tsp white stevia powder

Fold eggs into coconut mixture until well combined (you will lose most of the volume of the eggs)

Make 2-inch balls, place 2 inches apart, bake 10 minutes or until golden brown.

📖 More Information

Books

Anything by Thich Nhat Hanh

Biology of Belief by Bruce Lipton

Blink by Malcom Gladwell

Bringing Yoga to Life by Donna Farhi

The Detox Book by Bruce Fife

Dr. Mercola's Total Health by Dr. Joseph Mercola (Mercola.com is a good place to search for answers to health questions)

Herbal Medicine for Health and Well-Being by Laura Washington, ND

Home Enlightenment by Annie Bond

The Intention Experiment by Lynne McTaggart

Light on Yoga and *Light on Life* by BKS Iyengar

Meditations from the Mat by Rolf Gates

The Metabolic Typing Diet by William Wilcott and Trish Fahey

The Mindbody Prescription by John Sarno, MD

Minding the Body, Mending the Mind by Joan Borysenko, Ph.D.

Molecules of Emotion by Candace Pert, Ph.D. (or others by her)

Power of Now by Eckhart Tolle (or other books by him)

Psychology of Achievement by Brian Tracy (or others by him), highly recommended!

The Safe Shoppers Bible by David Steinman and Samuel Epstein

The 7 Habits of Highly Effective People and *The 8th Habit* by Stephen Covey

Tao of Healthy Eating by Bob Flaws

Total Renewal and *Spent* by Frank Lipman, MD

Movies

"What the Bleep Do We Know?"

Articles

76 Ways Sugar Can Ruin Your Health

The following is taken from a listing of some of sugar's metabolic consequences from a variety of medical journals and other scientific publications. The list "76 Ways Sugar Can Ruin Your Health" was compiled by Nancy Appleton, Ph.D., author of *Lick the Sugar Habit*.

Sugar can:

1. Suppress your immune system and impair your defenses against infectious disease

2. Upset the mineral relationships in your body: causes chromium and copper deficiencies and interferes with absorption of calcium and magnesium

3. Cause a rapid rise of adrenaline, hyperactivity, anxiety, difficulty concentrating and crankiness in children

4. Produce a significant rise in total cholesterol, triglycerides and bad cholesterol and a decrease in good cholesterol

5. Causes a loss of tissue elasticity and function

6. Feed cancer cells and has been connected with the development of cancer of the breast, ovaries, prostate, rectum, pancreas, biliary tract, lung, gallbladder and stomach

7. Increase fasting levels of glucose and can cause reactive hypoglycemia

8. Weaken eyesight

9. Cause many problems with the gastrointestinal tract including: an acidic digestive tract, indigestion, malabsorption in patients with functional bowel disease, increased risk of Crohn's disease and ulcerative colitis

10. Cause premature aging

11. Lead to alcoholism

12. Cause your saliva to become acidic, tooth decay and periodontal disease

13. Contribute to obesity

14. Cause autoimmune diseases such as: arthritis, asthma, multiple sclerosis

15. Greatly assist the uncontrolled growth of Candida Albicans (yeast infections)

16. Cause gallstones

17. Cause appendicitis

18. Cause hemorrhoids

19. Cause varicose veins

20. Elevate glucose and insulin responses in oral contraceptive users

21. Contribute to osteoporosis

22. Cause a decrease in your insulin sensitivity thereby causing an abnormally high insulin levels and eventually diabetes

23. Lower your Vitamin E levels

24. Increase your systolic blood pressure

25. Cause drowsiness and decreased activity in children

26. Increase advanced glycation end products (AGEs)(Sugar molecules attaching to and thereby damaging proteins in the body)

27. Interfere with your absorption of protein

28. Cause food allergies

29. Cause toxemia during pregnancy

30. Contribute to eczema in children

31. Cause atherosclerosis and cardiovascular disease

32. Impair the structure of your DNA

33. Change the structure of protein and cause a permanent alteration of the way the proteins act in your body

34. Make your skin age by changing the structure of collagen

35. Cause cataracts and nearsightedness

36. Cause emphysema

37. Impair the physiological homeostasis of many systems in your body

38. Lower the ability of enzymes to function

39. Increase the size of your liver by making your liver cells divide and it can increase the amount of liver fat

40. Increase kidney size and produce pathological changes in the kidney such as the formation of kidney stones

41. Damage your pancreas

42. Increase fluid retention

43. Compromise the lining of your capillaries

44. Make your tendons more brittle

45. Cause headaches, including migraines

46. Reduce the learning capacity, adversely affect school children's grades and cause learning disorders

47. Cause an increase in delta, alpha and theta brain waves which can alter your mind's ability to think clearly

48. Cause depression

49. Increase your risk of gout

50. Increase your risk of Alzheimer's disease

51. Cause hormonal imbalances such as: increasing estrogen in men, exacerbating PMS and decreasing growth hormone

52. Lead to dizziness

53. Increase free radicals and oxidative stress

54. Significantly increase platelet adhesion in patients with peripheral vascular disease

55. Can lead to a substantial decrease in gestation duration and is associated with a twofold increased risk for delivering a small-for-gestational-age (SGA) infant in pregnant adolescents

56. Be intoxicating, similar to alcohol

57. Can affect the amount of carbon dioxide produced when given to premature babies

58. Your body changes sugar into 2 to 5 times more fat in the bloodstream than it does starch

59. Promote excessive food intake in obese subjects

60. Worsen the symptoms of children with attention deficit hyperactivity disorder (ADHD)

61. Adversely affect urinary electrolyte composition

62. Slow down the ability of your adrenal glands to function

63. Have the potential of inducing abnormal metabolic processes in a normal healthy individual and to promote chronic degenerative diseases

64. Cut off oxygen to your brain when given I.V.s (intravenous feedings) of sugar water

65. Increases your risk of polio

66. Cause epileptic seizures in high doses

67. Cause high blood pressure in those with obesity

68. Induce cell death

69. Cause gum disease

70. Affect bowel movement patterns and regularity

71. Dehydrate newborns

72. In juvenile rehabilitation camps, when children were put on a low sugar diet, there was a 44 percent drop in antisocial behavior

73. Sugar intake is higher in people with Parkinson's disease

74. Sugar is an addictive substance

75. Decrease in sugar intake can increase emotional stability

76. In intensive care units: Limiting sugar saves lives

Soda and Your Health

- Phosphates present in soda (regular or diet) act to leech the calcium of the bones, therefore being a major contributing factor to osteoporosis.

- Regular soda contains anywhere between 38 and 50 grams of sugar per a 12 oz. can, if you're drinking a 32 oz. drink you get about 140 grams of sugar, that's about 13 teaspoons of sugar per a 12 oz. can. Regular soda provides between 150-180 calories per 12 oz. can. One can of regular pop per day contains the maximum recommended intake of sugar a day.

- Excessive intake of regular soda can contribute to excessive calorie consumption leading to obesity and/or a decreased intake of foods that have a high nutrient value leading to deficiencies. A recent paper has proposed that high fructose corn syrup (used to sweeten most soft drinks) has specific metabolic consequences that favored obesity, while other evidence shows soft drinks can cause sharp insulin responses.

- People who drink 3 or more sugary sodas daily have 62 percent more dental decay, fillings and tooth loss. But sugar isn't the only ingredient in soft drinks that causes tooth problems, it's actually the acids included in many popular sodas that are said to "eat" away enamel and make teeth more prone to cavities. Acid begins to dissolve tooth enamel in only 20 minutes. Because saliva helps neutralize acids and wash your teeth clean, the worst time to drink soda pop, ironically, is when you are very thirsty or dehydrated due to low levels of saliva.

- Since these drinks are acidic they also bathe the lining of the esophagus as they are swallowed.

Carbonated drinks cause burping and some reflux of the acidic gastric juices from the stomach into the esophagus which is a suspected culprit of the increase in incidence of esophageal cancer in recent years.

• Studies suggest that soda may be associated with an increased risk of developing kidney stones.

• The stimulant properties and dependence potential of caffeine in soda are well documented, as are their effects on children.

• Despite the logic that consuming fewer calories will produce weight loss, the evidence is very clear that using artificial sweeteners will cause a paradoxical effect and actually cause you to gain weight. Nearly a decade ago, studies were already revealing that artificial sweeteners can stimulate your appetite, increase carbohydrate cravings and stimulate fat storage and weight gain. These chemical cocktails may be a powerful contributing factor in the obesity epidemic many industrialized nations are now experiencing. In Chinese Medicine it is believed that the flavor is an important factor not the calories, so if it tastes sweet that will be the effect on the body so there are no free foods.

• Also, several studies have pointed out the link between sugar and increased rates of cancer. Soda is loaded with sugar, which not only feeds cancer but also throws off insulin levels, leading to damaging effects on your health. For these reasons alone, eliminating soda from your diet is an absolute necessity to maintaining optimal health. Normalizing your insulin levels is one of the most powerful physical actions you can take to improve your health and lower your risk of cancer along with other long-term chronic health conditions such as obesity and diabetes. Fortunately, it is also the variable most easily influenced by healthy eating and exercise.

• Sucralose and Aspartame can trigger or worsen:

  • Diabetes
  • Fibromyalgia
  • Irritable Bowel Syndrome
  • Chronic fatigue syndrome
  • Parkinson's disease
  • Alzheimer's disease
  • Brain tumors
  • Lymphoma
  • Birth defects
  • Multiple sclerosis
  • Epilepsy

weekly overhaul
clear goals, to succeed
(one day a week off)

Made in the USA
Charleston, SC
15 November 2010